RAMIEL N

CURE GUM DISEASE NATURALLY

Heal and Prevent Periodontal Disease and Gingivitis with Whole Foods

FOREWORD BY PERIODONTIST
ALVIN DANENBERG, DDS

Golden Child Publishing
Montpelier, Vermont

About the Photos of Weston A. Price, DDS

These photographs are currently in print as part of the updated 8th edition of the book Nutrition and Physical Degeneration published by the Price-Pottenger Nutrition Foundation. The usage here of photos taken by Weston A. Price, DDS does not represent an endorsement by the Price-Pottenger Nutrition Foundation, the copyright holders, for the accuracy of information presented by the author of this book.

For more information contact The Price-Pottenger Nutrition Foundation, which has owned and protected the documented research of Dr. Price since 1952. Photos and quotations are used with permission from The Price-Pottenger Nutrition Foundation, www.ppnf.org. Contact: info@ppnf.org ; 800-366-3748.

Golden Child Publishing, Inc.
32 Main St. 186
Montpelier, VT 05602

ISBN–13: 978-0-9820213-6-1
ISBN–10: 0-9820213-6-4

Printed and bound in the United States of America
For media appearance requests for Mr. Nagel contact: pr@curegumdisease.com
For wholesale orders contact Golden Child Publishing at:
orders@goldenchildpublishing.com
To order copies visit: www.curegumdisease.com
For suggestions or corrections contact: comments@curegumdisease.com

Editors: Katherine Czapp, Stickler Editing, sticklerediting.com
Sandrine Love, nourishingourchildren.org
Illustrations: Jocelyn Gardner, www.joss0ne.com
Interior Design: Janet Robbins, www.nwdpbooks.com

Advocating for Holistic Dental Health

Ramiel Nagel is an author and Dental Health Advocate. He advocates for the protection of consumers against invasive and unnecessary dental procedures. Important information about gum disease is not being shared or promoted by the mainstream dental profession at an extreme detriment to the consumer. The purpose of this book is to educate the consumer about vital withheld information concerning oral health.

Author's Disclaimer

Ramiel Nagel is not a dentist, periodontist, or other licensed health care practitioner. He is a consumer health advocate and educator. This book represents a minority opinion about the nature of gum disease and holistic treatments. It is an expression of free speech, and is intended for educational purposes only.

This book is not meant to be a replacement for treatment or a justification for declining the services of licensed dental care practitioners. Any application of the information in this book is done at the reader's own risk and discretion. Any individual with specific health problems or who is taking medications should consult his or her physician, dentist, or other licensed health care provider before following any advice presented in this book.

Neither Ramiel Nagel, nor Golden Child Publishing, Inc., shall have liability or responsibility to any person or entity with respect to loss, damage, or injury caused or alleged to be caused directly or indirectly by the information contained in this book. We assume no legal liability for errors, inaccuracies, omissions, or any inconsistency herein. We will however make corrections to information, based on evidence, as it is presented to us in a timely manner where possible. The information in this book does not replace the advice of a trained dentist or periodontist. Diseased states require medical supervision. The author is not a licensed health care professional and does not provide medical advice or consultation.

Contents

Forward

By Nutritional Periodontist Alvin H. Danenberg, DDS

I am a periodontist who has been treating gum disease for forty-one years. For the first thirty-five years of my career, like almost every other periodontist, I ignored nutrition, and I treated advanced gum disease with open flap surgery and everything else that went with it. The "everything else" included cutting with scalpels, placing bone grafts, using stitches, and prescribing antibiotics. Patients were not the happiest people because they had to endure discomfort during the healing process and the long-term results were somewhat questionable.

My colleagues and I had patients who came to us every six months for decades, followed the prescribed treatments, and occasionally had recurring gum disease. While we asked the fundamental question, "Why was this happening?", we did not understand the relationship of primal nutrition to the progression of gum disease.

In 2013, I learned about primal nutrition and the science that demonstrates that our poor diets—which lack nutrient-dense, whole foods—are damaging our gut and overall health. The result is degenerative and chronic diseases, including gum disease. Our primal ancestors hardly had gum disease because they only ate nutrient-dense, real foods. Today's modern meals consist of processed foods with additives and toxins. These so-called foods lack many of the essential nutrients our bodies need to survive and thrive. And when people do not get the nutrition needed by our bodies, individual cells suffer, and eventually organ systems suffer, and eventually the whole body including the mouth suffers.

Unfortunately, members of my profession have little knowledge of the importance of primal nutrition and its direct impact on our health. The science has been there, but unfortunately the majority of medical professionals have remained ignorant. I see my patients benefiting from primal nutrition, and I make sure that they all understand how to integrate healthy food choices as part of their periodontal treatment program so they get results that last.

I was searching in the dental world for others who were integrating primal nutrition with dental care. I found Ramiel's name and his book, *Cure Tooth Decay*. I made contact, read his book, and the rest is history. I was in for a treat when I first met Ramiel and I believe that you are in for a treat when you read this book. Our common ground has been nutrition and its effects on oral disease and healing. He and I began collaborating on a study I wanted to do in my offices for a select group of my patients to learn how nutrient-dense, real food supplements would affect the progression of gum disease. In this book, you will read about the significant positive results we obtained as well as many of Ramiel's eye-opening concepts.

Ramiel takes a sincere and critical look at how gum disease is treated in the U.S. today. Or should I say, how gum disease is mistreated? I think it is an injustice not to inform patients that there are nutritional solutions that prevent gum disease, which is a type of chronic disease. Proper nutrition could have prevented most gum disease problems we see today.

Ramiel will make some strong statements about my profession. He will make you think. His story is compelling, and he presents a life-changing formula to get your body healthy and thereby get your mouth healthy.

This is a book you must read. Pass it onto everyone you love and care about.

Alvin H. Danenberg, DDS
Periodontist of forty-one years
Specializing in evolutionary nutrition and laser treatment in Bluffton, South Carolina
www.drdanenberg.com

Introduction

The prospect of losing all of our teeth someday is a frightening thought. Yet as we age, we tend to lose more and more teeth with each passing decade. On average 25 percent of people in the United States over the age of sixty-five have no teeth at all because they have lost them not primarily due to dental caries, but to gum disease. This trend of tooth loss associated with advancing age is expected to continue to increase. Even people who have no teeth at all continue to suffer bone loss and degeneration of the mouth and jaw, making dentures uncomfortable, and requiring fittings for new dentures with unpleasant regularity. Without the benefit of our natural teeth, it is hard to savor and receive the delicious nourishment life has to offer.

The field of modern dentistry has got the perspective of dental care all wrong by only examining what is happening in the mouth while ignoring the rest of the body. This isolationist viewpoint entirely ignores the fact that our teeth and gums are connected to the rest of our bodies. The eyes are the window to the soul, and the mouth is a window into the inner condition of health and balance in the body. As a result of only looking at oral tissues, there is an over focus on fixing gum disease surgically with a cut, poison, and burn approach. The treatments can be painful and costly. After surgery there is not even a cosmetic improvement, as tissue has been excised and the gums will end up much lower on the gum line. In the long run, all of these conventional treatments might slow the disease process but they do not stop it. You are probably not going to hear from your dentist the truth that the long-term prognosis from gum surgeries is poor, seemingly because the business made from inserting dental implants when the surgical treatments fail and teeth are lost is far too profitable for the dental industry. As a result the patient is not informed about the expected results in advance.

However, the good news is that people have successfully cured their gum disease and stopped the destruction of teeth and bones by changing what they eat and consciously improving their diet. After all, it makes sense that what we eat will affect the tissues in our mouths.

Loose teeth, inflammation of oral tissues, pain from biting and chewing food, and tooth loss is pure suffering. Not being told by dental and health professionals that dental problems are primarily caused from a poor diet including too much sugar and too few vital nutrients allows this suffering to continue needlessly.

Curing gum disease is not just about healing your gums; it's about changing your life. It is about time that we stop giving up on ourselves, and on each other. Let me be forthcoming here: there is no "quick fix." It takes time, energy, and effort to make a real change to address the cause of gum disease.

This book is meant to challenge the entire complacent dental profession, to obliterate dogmatic and limiting beliefs, and to give you the power, evidence, and specific protocols and guidelines that you need to get to the core of gum disease and stop it permanently.

Once you read this book, the decision to cure gum disease naturally will be yours and yours alone. You will know how to navigate the treacherous waters of periodontal treatments and set your course straight to the goal so that you can keep your teeth for the rest of your life.

You Can Heal Gum Disease Naturally!

Healing gum disease requires us to open ourselves to new possibilities in life. Imagine that the sun is shining upon you, warming your body deeply. The sun is an outer expression of what lives in you: light, love, energy, and pure radiance. You suffer from gum disease because in some way your light has become dimmed. A dimmed inner light leads to living a diluted life, where the fullness and richness of life is not being completely received and experienced. Knowing that you can heal, opening your heart and mind to that possibility, and inviting in change is the most important step you can take toward healing gum disease.

How This Book Is Different from Other Books That Promise Natural Gum Disease Reversal

Many books about gum disease and much of the literature concerning gum disease imply that the cure for gum disease has already been found. But a deeper inquiry into the treatment models shows the same disempowering recommendations of surgery and anti-bacterial treatments. This book is a new inquiry into gum disease—its goal is to teach you the foundational causes of gum disease, and the changes required to stop the condition at the level of cause.

The point of this book is not to rehash the standard dental mantra that you have likely already heard about gum disease: that you should brush and floss daily, schedule dental cleanings twice a year, submit to deeper cleanings to eliminate calculus and plaque, and finally elect to undergo gum surgery if the deep cleaning fails to keep you healthy. The point of the book is to teach you how to cure gum disease naturally!

What You Can Expect When You Cure Gum Disease

The purpose of this book is to help you elevate the care of your oral health. As you will see for yourself from the evidence presented, the only sane approach for treating gum disease is to address its real cause: a poor diet and a lack of absorption of nutrients! The results you will get from making this choice are hard to predict because each and every person is so unique.

People who read this book and then apply the advice to their life can expect to learn specifically how to address the true cause of gum disease with practical steps. This would mean that over time you will no longer suffer from further inflammation, loss, and deterioration of your gums or jaw bones. Many of you who work diligently will keep your gums and the supporting tissues healthy for the rest of your life. You can substantially reduce the need for, or avoid completely: dentures, tooth implants, loose teeth, bleeding gums, gum infections near the tooth root, further gum recession, bone loss, and the seemingly never ending treadmill of unnecessary dental procedures for your gums.

In the case of gingivitis, many readers should find that following the advice in this book over a period of weeks or months will significantly improve or completely reverse the condition.

Healing periodontal disease takes time. You may see some results in as little as two weeks, but expect at least two to three months, depending on the situation, to really slow down or stop the condition in its tracks solely with diet. It can take about one year provided you have made significant positive lifestyle and dietary changes for X-rays to show an improvement in bone density.

The primary cause of gum disease is nutritional, but ongoing destructive forces in the mouth caused by bite imbalances, or an excess condition of infection in the gums, can significantly impair or completely block the healing process. Correcting a problem with the bite may require a night guard and an advanced state of infection might require professional services of a periodontist. In Chapter 9 on dentistry, I will help you understand the least invasive procedures available that can support your healing process. But the point here is that for some of you, the best results will happen with some additional structural care that can support the healing process. I will provide you with information on the treatments available so you can feel clear and empowered on how you want to heal your gums.

About Ramiel Nagel, Author of *Cure Gum Disease Naturally*

I grew up in the south part of the San Francisco Bay Area in a typical suburban neighborhood. I went to college at the University of California Santa Cruz and I found myself longing for something more fulfilling than academic learning. In the freedom of the redwood trees and the somewhat relaxed atmosphere, I found my desire to learn about myself. I became a devoted hatha yoga student, and soon found that my yoga practice was far more satisfying than academic learning. I graduated with a B.A. in legal studies.

Once I finished at the University, I found myself lost in the world, not really fitting in. I signed up for a program that taught energy medicine which was based in a system of body-oriented psychotherapy called Core Energetics. In this self-search, I started to let go of past attachments, and connect with forgotten feelings. As my mind and emotions became more clear, I felt like I had something good to offer the world, but I did not know what it was.

I many times aligned myself and prayed to be of service to others. After my first daughter was born and began suffering from tooth decay, I delved into health research. I found that I had a knack for making sense of it all in a way that it seemed like others had missed. My desire to help others and share what I have learned has resulted in three books:

Cure Tooth Decay—www.curetoothdecay.com
Healing our Children—www.healingourchildren.net

And the book you are reading right now. Currently my family and I are planning to start a holistic learning center for children and adults, along with a farm, on the East Coast.

1 Understanding Gum Disease so You Can Heal

Right now I encourage you to take the first step toward healing gum disease. And that step is to make the choice to heal. I want you to heal, and so I align with this purpose. If you will, take a moment and align with your own personal goal for healing gum disease. Imagine your teeth feeling strong and firmly implanted in healthy gums. Imagine yourself enjoying life and feeling good and nourished. Start healing gum disease by changing how you think and imagining a better future for yourself. Do this now!

By working with people to heal their gum disease I have found that success is determined before you begin. For those of you who align with and open yourselves to a positive energy stream, a good vibration, or a deep soul current toward health, will be the ones to succeed. For those of you who feel closed, resistant, doubtful, and unwilling to do the work that it takes to heal, you will be the ones who usually fail. But don't worry if you are a habitual skeptic, or disbeliever. I am skeptical, too. Skepticism can be healthy. And if you've been burned too many times by false hopes and painful treatments, then naturally it is hard to be optimistic. But if your skepticism is a tool of resistance and stagnation which blocks you from taking positive action, then your skepticism will be a hindrance on your path to recovery.

In order for you to succeed and understand gum disease, I urge you to give yourself the time you need and deserve to understand gum disease thoroughly. If your goal is simply to rush past the slow and deliberate decay of your body, then your odds of successfully healing this condition decrease quite a bit. You cannot succeed if you hurriedly try to eliminate the disease from your mind, so that you can move on to the next "more important" thing. Your goal if you want to succeed must be to face your reality, so you can do something about it.

Readers who merely skim through this book will miss out on understanding the thought process behind the recommendations, and as a result will end up confused and unsure of themselves. The purpose here is to educate and encourage an inner change of awareness about health for the reader. The aim is for you to begin to ask the right questions and become an authority and an advocate for your own health.

This book is meant to bring you closer to the rules of the natural world so you can understand how the effect of gum disease was created. I want you to find your own inner wisdom and authority when it comes to gum health. The words and message here are not meant to squash, suppress, or replace what you know and feel to be true. This is not meant to supplant your own wisdom, but rather to enhance it.

Do not take what I write here on faith; that is not my goal. Review the evidence and allow it to help you draw your own conclusions as to the real nature of gum disease and how to treat it. I believe that when you see some of the facts that have been hidden and not shared, that you will more easily be able to come to your own educated decision about what is best for you.

What Is Gum Disease?

A brief anatomy review is important to help define and clarify the condition of gum disease. **Gum disease is caused by a deficiency of nutrients in your body which for some people results in inflammation and bone loss in your periodontium.**

The periodontium consists of four components:

- Gum tissue which is the pink skin in your mouth and specifically around your teeth.

Anatomy of the Periodontium

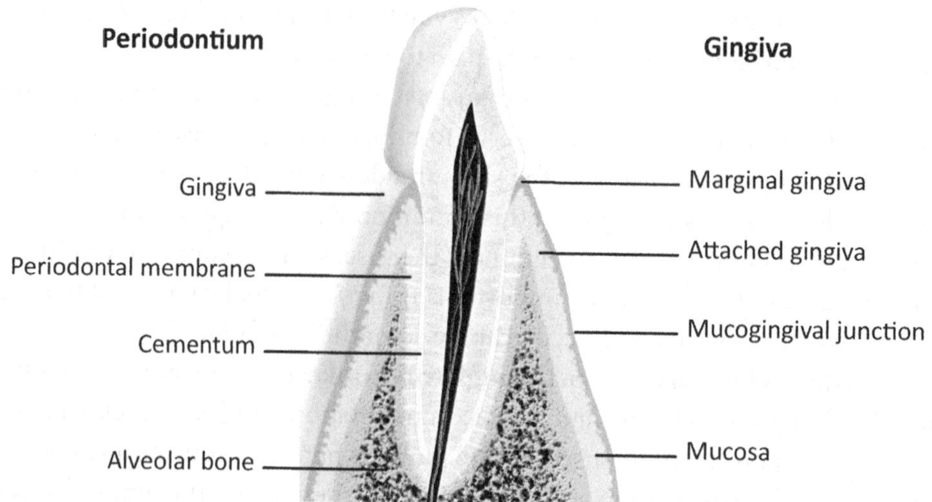

- The periodontal ligament, which is the matrix of micro cartilaginous strands that secure the teeth into the socket similar to the way cables hold up a suspension bridge. The periodontal ligament is sandwiched between the cementum and the alveolar bone. The periodontal ligament actually suspends the tooth in the socket, so that it can depress, flex, rotate, and move in ways to accommodate biting and chewing forces without damaging the tooth or the alveolar bone.
- The cementum is the outer layer of the tooth which is below the gum line, which through the periodontal ligaments connects your gum tissue to the alveolar bone.
- The alveolar bone is the part of the maxilla (palate) and mandible (jaw) bone that contains the socket that holds the tooth in place.

Gingivitis

Gingival means pertaining to the gums and *itis* means inflammation. Gingivitis means inflammation of the gum tissues without loss of connective tissue attachment.

The true cause of this condition is a nutritional deficiency resulting in tissue inflammation.

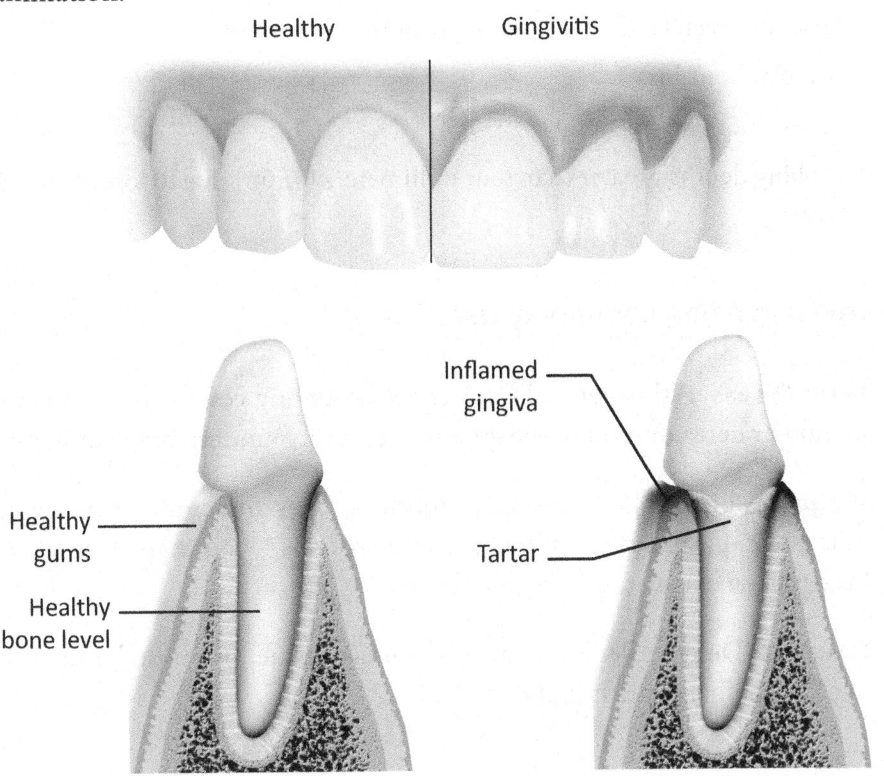

Gingivitis Symptoms

- ☐ Red or reddish-blue gums
- ☐ Swollen tissue at the gingival margin
- ☐ Bleeding upon gentle probing[1], normal brushing or flossing.

Periodontitis (also called gum disease, periodontal disease, and formerly known as pyorrhea)

Peri means around, odont means tooth, and itis means inflammation. Periodontitis means inflammation of the area around your tooth. Periodontitis is the progressive loss of the alveolar bone around the teeth. Periodontitis involves gum tissue inflammation at sites where there has been a consistent detachment of connective tissue from the cementum, the base of the gum has migrated away from its apex, and **bone loss** can be detected by X-ray. Periodontitis also involves the presence of bleeding on probing, deep pockets, recession, and tooth mobility[2]. Its real cause is demineralization of tissues and bones from nutritional deficiencies and the resulting infection and loss of the maxilla and mandible bones.

Periodontal (Gum Disease) Symptoms

- ☐ Space between teeth where gums are normally present
- ☐ Alveolar bone loss
- ☐ Excess tooth mobility
- ☐ Probing depths greater than four millimeters (4mm) due to loss of connective tissue[3].

Understanding Commonly Used Terms

Gum Disease: This general term can refer to any condition of inflammation or deterioration of the gum tissue or surrounding tissue or bone.

Plaque: A biofilm that adheres to tooth surfaces and contains bacteria, saliva, calcium and phosphorous, fat and proteins.[5] Plaque and not calculus has been correlated with gum disease.[6]

Calculus: Dental calculus is calcified dental plaque, composed primarily of calcium phosphate mineral salts.[7]

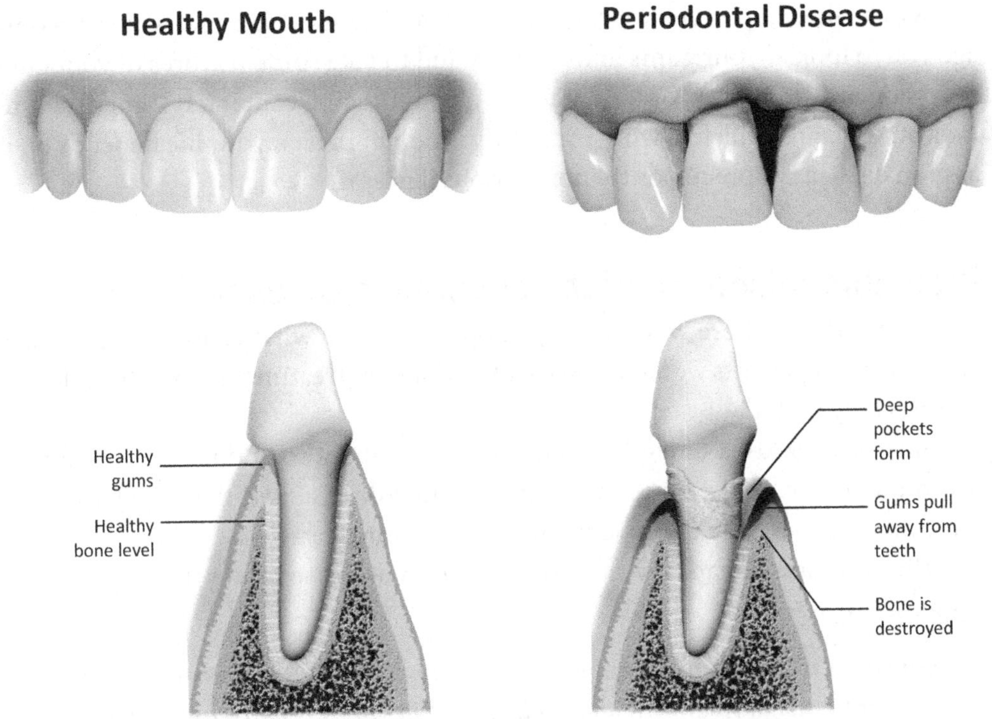

Healthy Mouth **Periodontal Disease**

Healthy gums
Healthy bone level

Deep pockets form
Gums pull away from teeth
Bone is destroyed

Moderate periodontal disease is defined as having at least two teeth with interproximal (in between teeth) attachment loss of four millimeters or more OR at least two teeth with five millimeters or more of pocket depth at interproximal sites. The prevalence of moderate periodontitis in the U.S. is 30 percent of adults. The prevalence of moderate periodontitis increases with age with those over sixty-five years the most affected.[4]

Severe periodontal disease is defined as having at least two teeth with interproximal (in between teeth) attachment loss of six millimeters or more AND at least one tooth with five millimeters or more of pocket depth at interproximal sites. Severe periodontitis was estimated to occur in 8.5 percent of U.S. adults over thirty years of age; that's more than twenty million people.

Stop and Take a Good Look at Your Gum Disease

The healing process begins when you fully own, or embody your suffering. Loose teeth, inflammation of oral tissues, pain from biting and chewing food, and losing teeth, is suffering. Not knowing what to do about this disease as it progresses and worsens compounds the suffering. Take a moment right now to notice how you feel about your experience of gum disease.

As a further step of acknowledgment of your health situation, I would encourage you to look at your gums in the mirror and to take some pictures of your gum recession, inflammation, or loose teeth with your digital camera. It's important to look at, see, and really feel what your body is doing. In fact, your life depends on it as gum disease is a precursor to more serious illnesses.

Profitable Misconceptions about Gum Disease

Before the 1970s, there was a variety of opinions as to what caused gum disease, and as a result, patients would receive widely different treatments from the different dentists they visited.

Since the 1970s, a unified message has been taught to and by the dental profession: that bacterial plaque causes periodontal disease and that regular plaque removal is the best way to prevent and treat the disease.[8]

The American Academy of Periodontology website offers this explanation for gum disease:

> *Gingivitis is often caused by inadequate oral hygiene. Gingivitis is reversible with professional treatment and good oral home care. . . .* ***Untreated gingivitis can advance to periodontitis.*** *With time, plaque can spread and grow below the gum line.* ***Toxins produced by the bacteria*** *in plaque irritate the gums.* ***The toxins stimulate a chronic inflammatory response*** *in which the body in essence turns on itself, and the tissues and bone that support the teeth are broken down and destroyed. Gums separate from the teeth, forming pockets (spaces between the teeth and gums) that become infected.*[9]

Summary on Currently Believed Gum Disease Theory

Poor oral hygiene ▸ Gingivitis
Untreated gingivitis ▸ Excess bacterial toxins in plaque
Excess bacterial toxins over time ▸ Gum disease (periodontitis)

All of us who have been in a dental chair have been told that mantra so often that most of us believe it to be true. But the truth is that there is no consensus about bacteria as the cause of gum disease.

A 1997 article in the *Journal of the American Academy of Periodontology* states there are more than three hundred types of bacteria in the mouth, but *"very few of these bacteria cause systemic infection in healthy individuals."* Furthermore our *"innate host defense system,"* constantly monitors, and *"prevents bacterial intrusion."*[10] What this means is that there is always a variety of bacteria in our mouth, and our body usually prevents the few "bad" bacteria from becoming too prevalent.

The concept of a "host defense system"—meaning our body's ability to monitor and control bacterial infections—is also well accepted in the field of periodontology. In 2005 the American Academy of Periodontology concluded that only 20 percent of periodontal disease can be attributed to bacteria and cited host response as the key factor in gum disease.[11]

This conclusion matters because the concept of our body's ability to protect itself and maintain health, what the literature refers to as *host response,* is the key variable which determines why some people have gum disease and others do not. Periodontal researchers have acknowledged and accepted that periodontal disease is a systemic disease focused on the body's reaction to bacteria, and is therefore a "multifactorial, complex disease."[12]

What's more, researchers have documented the episodic and periodic nature of gum disease. With *chronic periodontitis,* periods of "rapid progression" are followed by long periods of "remission."[13] This simply would seem to acknowledge that gum disease can go into remission by itself, although the modern dental industry does not seem to know why. The systemic nature of gum disease is further illustrated by aggressive periodontitis, the term for fast acting gum recession that occurs primarily in young people during times of rapid growth. This is not caused by bacteria, but by the rapid depletion of vitamins and minerals caused by growth spurts.

Gingivitis Does Not Inevitably Lead to Periodontitis

The currently accepted theory of the cause of gum disease holds that untreated gingivitis always leads to periodontal disease. However, scientific evidence does not support that claim. Indeed, an American Academy of Periodontology position paper cites research dating back to the 1980s that proves "relatively few sites with gingivitis go on to develop periodontitis."[14]

A three-year study on gingivitis also found no obvious signs that gingivitis progressed to periodontal disease and went so far as to say, *"the subjects were relatively resistant to periodontitis."*[15] Furthermore, receiving professional dental cleanings every six months did not eliminate gingivitis.[16]

Gingivitis has also been found without the presence of plaque and without a greater than normal bacterial presence.[17]

While the research says that gingival sites do not go on to develop into full periodontal disease, there is a correlation between the illnesses. As we will see in Chapter 3, they have a similar underlying cause.

During 2009–2010, a large government survey showed how widespread gum disease is, and 45 percent of adults aged 45–64 had moderate and severe gum disease.[18]

As people age, they succumb to more and more gum disease. As we age we also lose more teeth. Not including wisdom teeth the average 20 to 39-year-old is missing 1 tooth, the average 40 to 49-year-old 3.5 teeth, and those aged 60 and over are missing 8 teeth primarily as a result of gum disease.

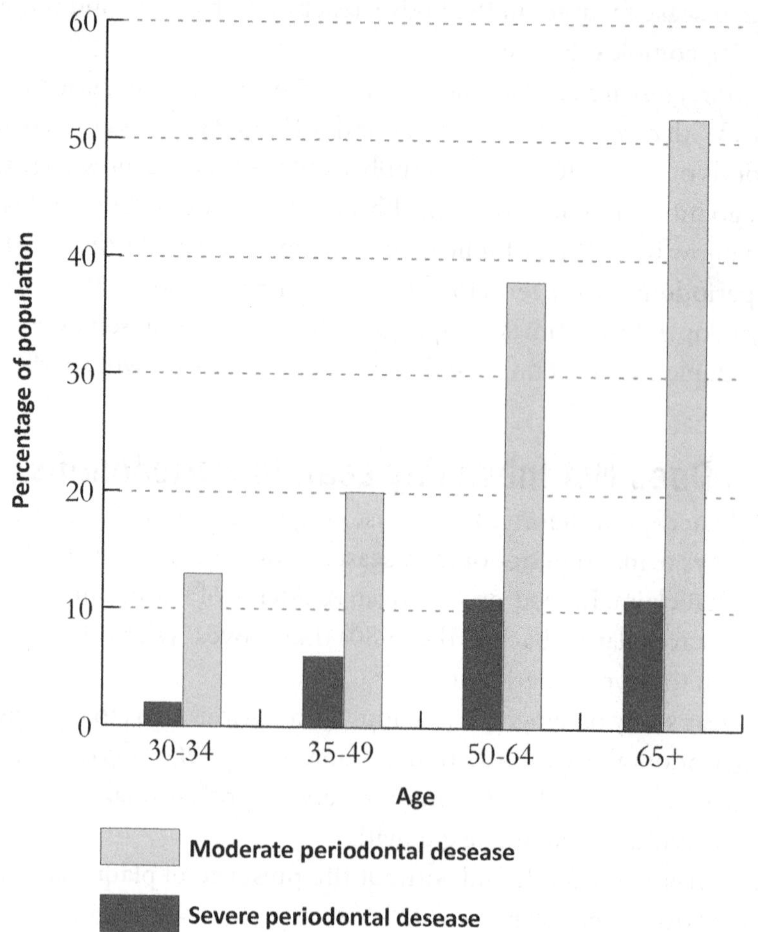

A More Accurate Picture of Gum Disease

In 2010, the authoritative *Periodontal Disease and Overall Health: A Clinician's Guide written* by dental professors and researchers published a more accurate picture on the cause of gum disease:

Now as a result of extensive research, it has been shown that periodontal disease is initiated by plaque, but the severity and progression of the disease is determined by the host response to the bacterial biofilm.[19] (Emphasis added.)

In the book, they go on to state that people with gingivitis might have severe plaque and calculus deposits, but that this won't necessarily lead to gum disease. Meanwhile, some people have excellent oral hygiene, without any of the obvious plaque or calculus deposits, and despite this they have severe gum disease with large pockets, loose teeth, and loss of teeth.[20] They conclude based on these observations that, ***"the host response to the bacterial challenge,*** presented by subgingival plaque, is the important determinant of disease severity."[21] (Emphasis added.)

These are two very different concepts about gum disease. The currently purported theory focuses on oral hygiene and bacterial toxins, while a more accurate and scientifically verified theory is that gum disease is primarily about the host response and how the body reacts to certain conditions. These two very different models about gum disease might and do lead to very different treatment approaches and results.

Summary of a More Accurate Theory as to the Cause of Gum Disease

Our body's response to the presence of plaque determines if we develop gum disease.

Positive host response with no plaque or calculus ▸ Healthy gums
Positive host response with severe plaque and calculus ▸ Gingivitis but not gum disease
Negative host response even with good hygiene ▸ Severe gum disease

Compare this more accurate theory with what the dental associations and dentists are teaching us today:

Summary on Currently Believed Gum Disease Theory

Poor oral hygiene ▸ Gingivitis
Untreated gingivitis ▸ Excess bacterial toxins in plaque
Excess bacterial toxins over time ▸ Gum disease (periodontitis)

Are we to believe that the 38.5 percent of the adult population with moderate to severe gum disease does not take adequate care of their teeth and gums? Or should we ask what other factors might influence our body, its response to bacteria, its production of plaque, and the development of this disease?

Let's start with a focused look at a primary determinant of your body's response to bacteria—the food we eat.

Summary of Key Points

- ☐ Health is your responsibility; your alignment and intention around health make a difference in your ability to cure gum disease.
- ☐ Gingivitis is reversible gum inflammation that does not increase with age.
- ☐ Periodontitis (gum disease) is bone loss in the jaw that is cyclical in nature and gets worse over time with age. It is regulated by host response.
- ☐ The field of dentistry focuses on the removal of plaque and the destruction caused by bacteria and it does not inform people clearly that the consensus of periodontal science is that your body's response to the plaque known as the "host response" is what really matters.

2 Improper Nutrition Is the Cause of Gum Disease

Many surveys on ancient skulls show that "primitive" humans were, with only a few exceptions, largely free of tooth decay and gum disease.[1] This is because traditional societies have benefited from an accumulation of wisdom over countless generations of how to live and reproduce with robust health.[2] If they did not know how to produce healthy bodies and healthy teeth and gums for generation after generation, then their society or population group would not have survived.

Weston A. Price, DDS, the first research director of the National Dental Association (now known as the American Dental Association, or ADA), suspected from observing the declining dental and overall health of his patients in Cleveland, Ohio, that something was fundamentally wrong with the way we live in modern society. Something was causing increased incidence of tooth decay and gum disease and causing a decline in general health among all ages of patients. Dr. Price's research was spurred by the loss of his only son, Donald, to the complications of an infected root canal that he had placed himself.[3]

In order to gain insights and satisfy his wish to learn more, he decided to travel around the world in the 1930s to study primitive cultures enjoying optimal physical and mental health. During his travels he not only found populations displaying healthy teeth and gums, but he was also able to observe the sharp decline in health experienced by previously healthy native peoples once they came into contact with what Dr. Price referred to as the "displacing foods of modern commerce." That term refers to industrially produced food products rather than real food. Through his words and photographs Dr. Price's landmark book, *Nutrition and Physical Degeneration,* proves that our modern food and lifestyle changes are the primary cause of physical degeneration, with one result being gum disease.

The Healthy People of the Loetschental, Switzerland

In 1931 and 1932, Dr. Price traveled to the remote Loetschental in the Swiss Alps. The people of the valley lived in harmony with nature, which resulted in a seemingly peaceful existence. Dr. Price wrote of the superior character and health of these people and the sublime lands of the isolated valleys in the remote Swiss Alps:

> *They have neither physician nor dentist because they have so little need for them; they have neither policeman nor jail, because they have no need for them.*[4]

This harmony was also evident in the production of food:

> *While the cows spend the warm summer on the verdant knolls and wooded slopes near the glaciers and fields of perpetual snow, they have a period of high and rich productivity of milk... This cheese contains the natural butter fat and minerals of the splendid milk and is* ***a virtual storehouse of life*** *for the coming winter.*[5] *(Emphasis added.)*

Reverend John Siegen, pastor of the only church in the valley at the time Price visited, told him about the divine characteristics of butter and cheese made from the milk of the grazing cows:

> *He told me that they recognize the presence of Divinity in the life-giving qualities of the butter made in June when cows have arrived for pasturage near the glaciers. He gathers the people together to thank the kind* ***Father*** *for evidence of his* ***Being*** *in the life-giving qualities of butter and cheese when the cows eat the grass near the snow line... The natives of the valley are able to recognize the superior quality of their June butter, and, without knowing exactly why,* ***pay it due homage.***[6] *(Emphasis added.)*

It was neither good genes nor luck that kept these isolated Swiss in superb health, but rather, it was how they lived and honored their food. Dr. Price continues:

> *One immediately wonders if there is not something in the life-giving vitamins and minerals of the food that builds not only great physical structures within which their souls reside, but builds minds and hearts capable of a higher type of manhood in which the material values of life are made secondary to individual character.*[9]

These healthy people are role models for us for living in health and relative peace. It is this way of being that has become lost in the modern world of convenience and fast "food." It is a result of our fall from grace. By sensing and revering the holy nature of food, ancient cultures enjoyed vibrant health. In exchange for their reverence of the life-giving vital force, especially of that in the summer milk and the cheese and butter made from it, the isolated Swiss received health, vigor, vitality, and peace.

Nutrition of the People in the Loetschental

The native Alpine Swiss diet consisted primarily of soured rye bread and summer cheese—the latter consumed in a portion about as large as the slice of bread but not as thick, which was eaten with fresh milk of goats or cows. Meat was eaten once a week and smaller portions of butter, vegetables, and barley were consumed regularly. Soup from animal bones was consumed regularly.

Diet of Healthy Indigenous People in the Swiss Alps[10]

Calories	Food	Fat-Soluble Vitamins	Calcium	Phosphorus
800	Rye Bread	Low	0.07	0.46
400	Milk	High	0.68	0.53
400	Cheese	Very High	0.84	0.62
100	Butter	Very High	0.00	0.00
100	Barley	Low	0.00	0.03
100	Vegetables	Low	0.06	0.08
100	Meat	Medium	0.00	0.12
2000		**Very High**	**1.76**	**1.84**

Immunity to Tooth Decay

The root of poor nutrition affects different people differently; some will develop gum disease, others will suffer tooth decay, and a few unlucky ones will endure both. Because of the similar cause (lack of nutrients), the immunity to tooth decay is still important to look at because it demonstrates how healthy these people were. In a study of 4,280 teeth of the children in these high valleys, only 3.4 percent were found to have been attacked by tooth decay. In Loetschental, 0.3 percent of all teeth were affected with tooth decay.[11]

Isolated Swiss Alps Children Were Remarkably Healthy

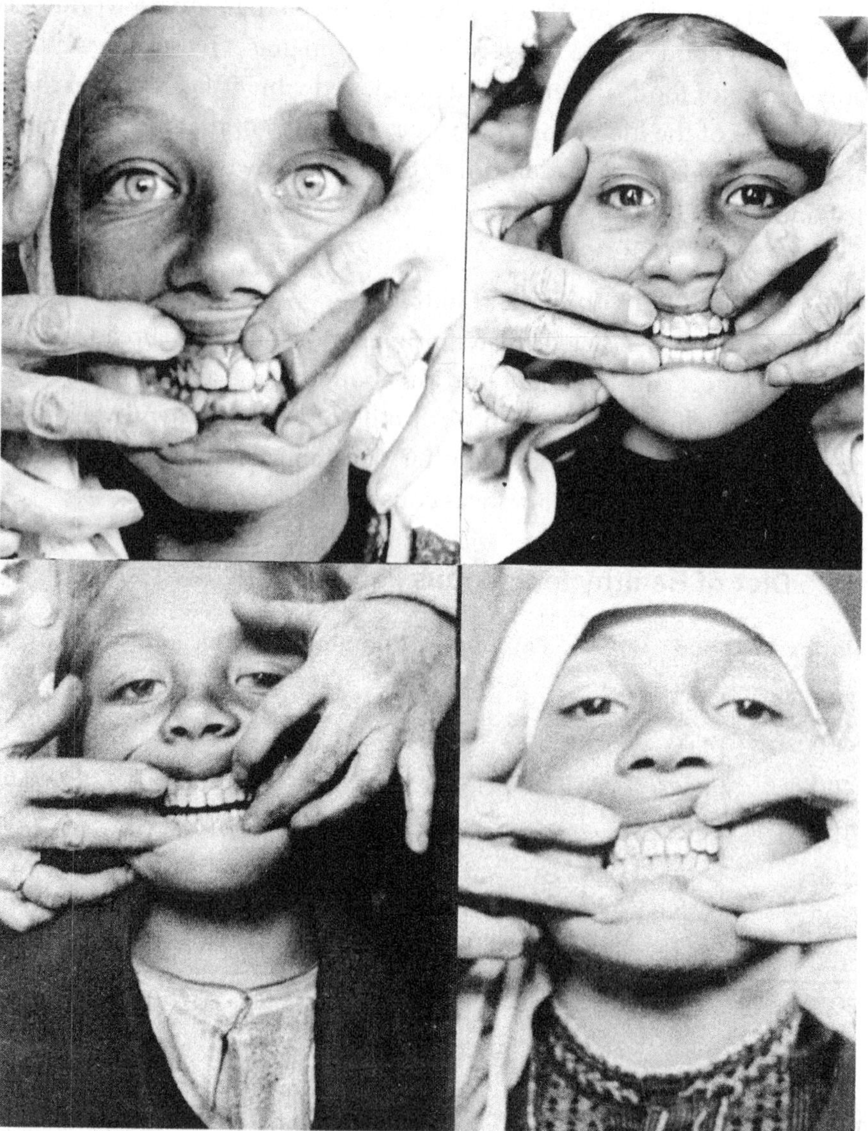

Normal design of face and dental arches when adequate nutrition is provided for both the parents and the children. Note the well-developed nostrils.[7] *(Original caption.)*

Modern Swiss Children Have Lost Their Dental Health

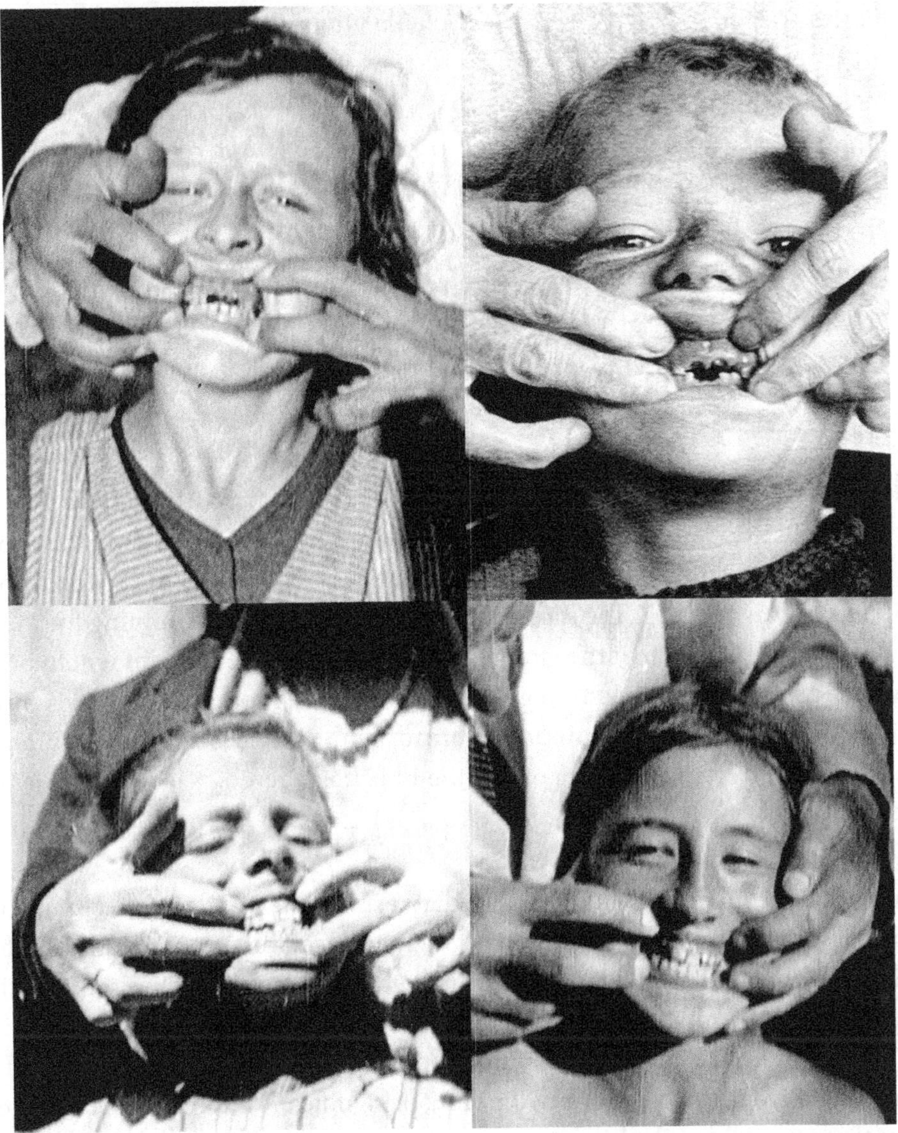

In the modernized districts of Switzerland tooth decay is rampant. The girl, upper left, is sixteen and the one to the right is younger. They use white bread and sweets liberally. The two children below have very badly formed dental arches with crowding of the teeth. This deformity is not due to heredity.[8] (Original caption.)

Nutrient-Displacing, Poor Health Causing Diet of Modern Swiss[12]

Calories	Food	Fat-Soluble Vitamins	Calcium	Phosphorus
1000	White Bread	Low	0.11	0.35
400	Jam, Honey, Sugar, Syrup	Low	0.05	0.08
100	Chocolate and Coffee	Low	0.02	0.07
100	Milk	High	0.17	0.13
100	Canned Vegetables	Low	0.08	0.08
100	Meat	Medium	0.01	0.11
100	Vegetable Fat	Low	0.00	0.00
100	Butter (dairy)	High	0.00	0.00
2000		**Low**	**0.44**	**0.82**

Modern Swiss Were Losing Their Health and Teeth

In the 1930s, tooth decay was a major problem for school children in the modern parts of Switzerland. Depending on the location, between 85-100 percent of the population was affected. The local health director advised sun tanning for the children as it was believed that the vitamins produced from the sunlight would prevent tooth decay. However, this strategy did not work. The modern-living Swiss no longer ate their native diets of soured rye bread, summer cheese, summer butter, and fresh goat or cow milk, and as a result, their health suffered.

The Nutrition of the Modern Swiss

Foods that the modern-living Swiss ate that resulted in poor dental health included white-flour products, marmalades, jams, canned vegetables, confections, and fruits. All of these devitalized foods were transported to the area. Only limited supplies of vegetables were grown locally.

While there are several differences between the modern industrial diet and isolated native diets, there are two points of significant interest. When you compare these two tables, the key nutrient differences between the diets are not related to rye bread versus white bread. Rather, five hundred calories of the modern diet comes from sweets and chocolate which are high in sugar and low in fat-soluble vitamins and minerals. These products replaced cheese and milk which were dense sources of minerals and fat-soluble vitamins.

Here is an interesting observation from Dr. Price of some of the modern Swiss:

We studied some children here whose parents retained their primitive methods of food selection, and without exception those who were immune to dental caries were eating a distinctly different food from those with high susceptibility to dental caries.[13]

Immunity to Tooth Decay

Of 2,065 teeth that Dr. Price analyzed in one study of modern Swiss, 25.5 percent had been attacked by tooth decay and many teeth had become infected.[14]

Real Milk Has Been Wrongly Vilified

Unfortunately in today's world, the once profoundly honored cow's milk—unpasteurized and grass-fed—which has brought health to people across the globe for thousands of years, is being attacked by our own state and federal governments. This whole, vital food has become an enemy of the state. When you and your friends and family reconnect with real food, you reconnect with the goodness of life. In this state, boundaries dissolve, and enemies become friends.

The Healthy Eskimos

In 1933 Dr. Price visited the Eskimos in the far reaches of Alaska to document how dietary changes were affecting their health.

Dr. Price wrote that indigenous Eskimos were free of both gum disease and tooth decay:

Many primitive peoples not only retain all of their teeth, many of them to an old age, but also have a healthy flesh supporting these teeth. This has occurred in spite of the fact that the [natives] have not had dentists to remove the deposits and no means for doing so for themselves. Note particularly the teeth of the Eskimos. The teeth are often worn nearly to the gum line and yet the gum tissue has not receded. Many of these primitive groups were practically free from the affection which we have included in the general term of pyorrhea or gingivitis.

Pyorrhea is a now outdated term for gum disease. Pyo means pus in Greek, and rrhea means flow or discharge. Pyorrhea refers to the discharge of pus around the gums.

Healthy Eskimos on Their Native Diet

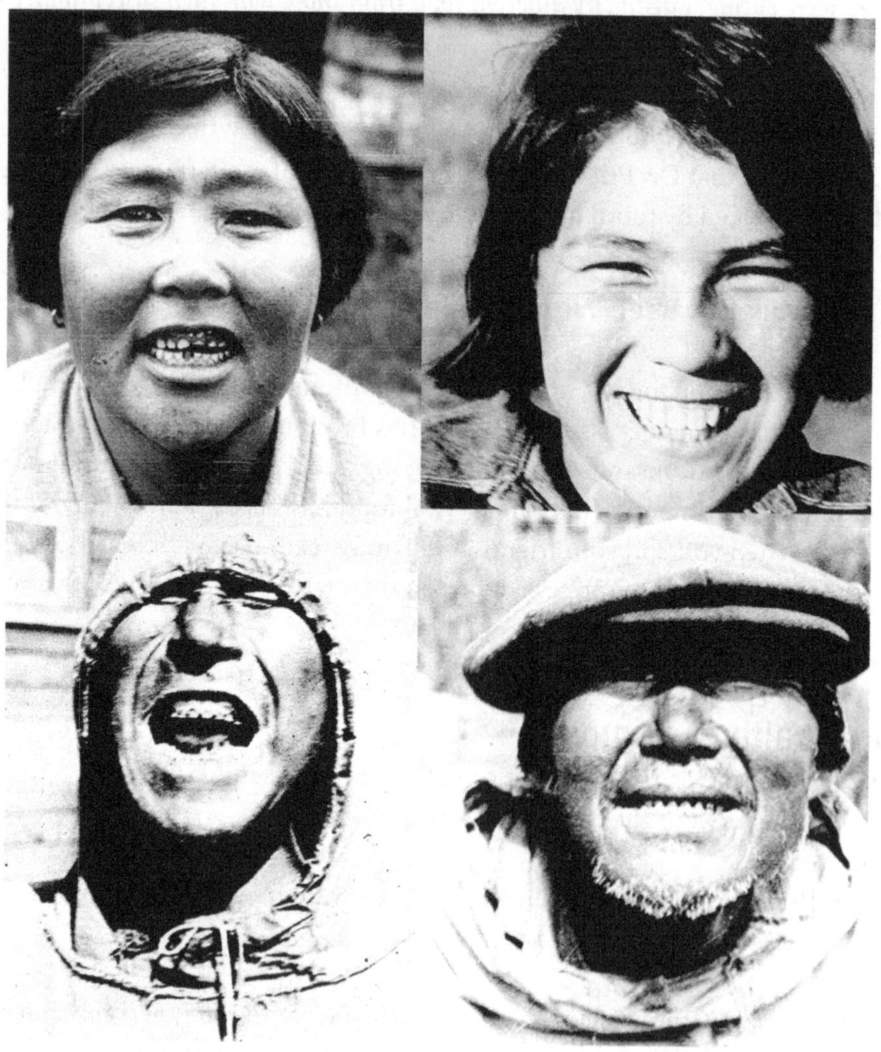

Typical native Alaskan Eskimos. Note the broad faces and broad arches and no dental caries (tooth decay). Upper left, woman has a broken lower tooth. She has had twenty-six children with no tooth decay. [15] (Original Caption)

When Eskimos Changed Their Diet They Suffered from Tooth Decay and Gum Disease

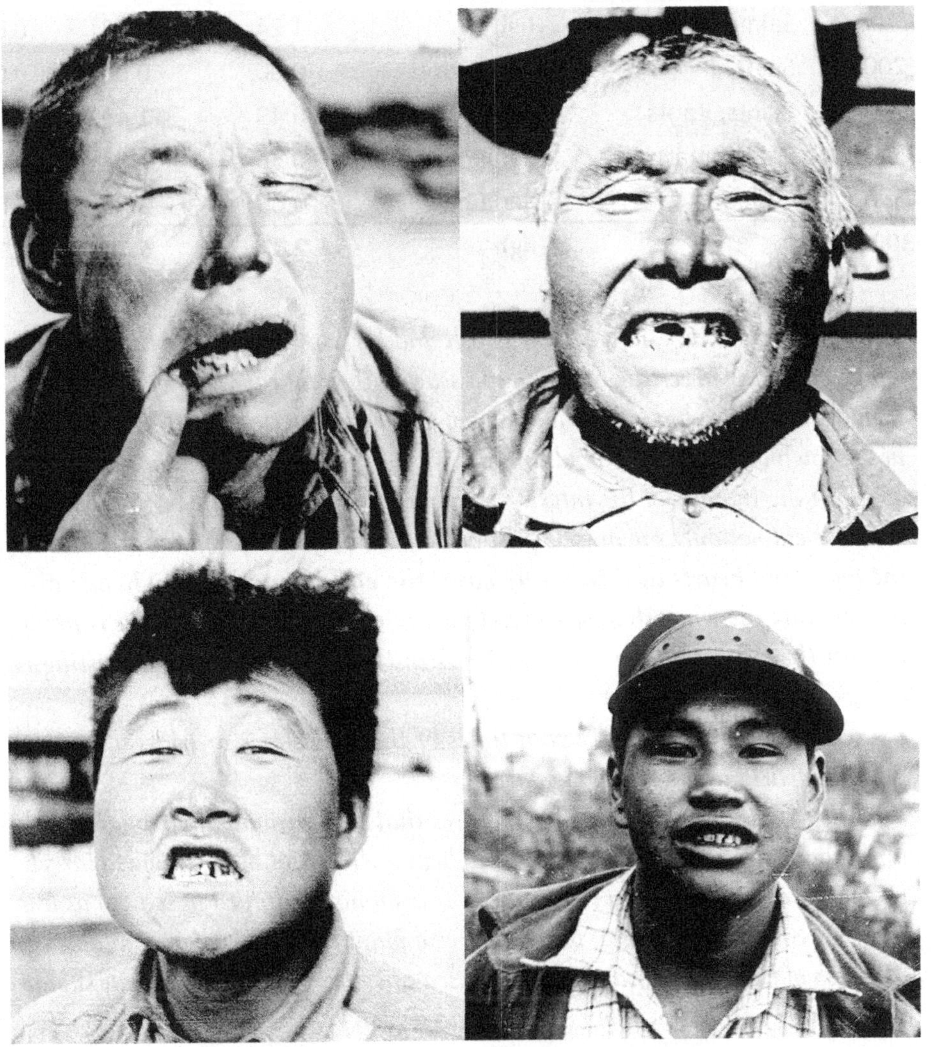

When the primitive Alaskan Eskimos obtain the white man's foods, dental caries become active. Pyorrhea also often becomes severe. In many districts dental service cannot be obtained and suffering is acute and prolonged.[21] (Original caption.)

When these adult Eskimos exchange their foods for our modern foods, they often have very extensive tooth decay and suffer severely.[22]

Traditional Diet of Healthy Indigenous Eskimos[16]

Calories	Food	Fat-Soluble Vitamins	Calcium	Phosphorus	Iron
1700	Salmon	High	1.24	2.68	0.05
200	Seal Oil	Very High	0.00	0.00	0.00
100	Plants, Roots	Low	0.49	1.40	0.04
500	Sea Animals	Medium	0.36	1.02	0.01
500	Caribou	Medium	0.05	0.60	0.00
3000		**High**	**2.14**	**5.70**	**0.10**

> *The bulk of their diet, however, was fish and large animal life of the sea from which they selected certain organs and tissues with great care and wisdom. These included the inner layer of skin of one of the whale species, which has recently been shown to be very rich in vitamin C.*[17]
>
> *Like the Indians of the interior who live on the animal life of the land the Eskimos eat not only the muscle part of fish and other forms of aquatic life but the livers and hearts* ***and in many cases the edible parts of the head;*** *also the milt and roe when these are present as is the case when the fish are running toward their spawning grounds which is the time the principal harvesting is done.*[18] *(Emphasis added.)*
>
> *[Eskimos] also use at certain times of the year stems or roots of certain plants, particularly the growing parts.*[19]
>
> *The severity of their weather requires that they provide their bodies with large quantities of fuel for production of heat... This would be provided largely by the stored smoked dried red salmon. This salmon is dipped in seal oil as it is eaten... Small quantities of parts of several plants are used when available... The flesh of walrus, seal, caribou, moose, sea cow, and occasionally whale should be a regular part of the menu according to season.*[20]

Dr. Price found that, time and time again, when *"blighted by the touch of modern civilization"*[23] with our foods of commerce, the once robust native person *"withers and dies."*[24]

In each example of native peoples from around the globe that Dr. Price visited, manufactured foods of industry caused the loss of pristine health when they replaced and displaced the traditional foods of the area. These modern foods included large amounts of white flour and sweeteners such as sugar, jams, and syrups, as well as sweetened goods and confections, canned fruits, canned vegetables,

The Modern Diet of Eskimos That Causes Tooth Decay and Gum Disease[25]

Calories	Food	Fat-Soluble Vitamins	Calcium	Phosphorus
1200	Bannock Bread (white flour)	Low	0.13	0.42
1200	Jam, Sugar, Syrup	Low	0.05	0.08
100	Chocolate and Coffee	Low	0.02	0.07
300	Meat	Medium	0.03	0.33
100	Vegetables	Low	0.06	0.08
100	Vegetable Fats	Low	0.00	0.00
3000		**Low**	**0.39**	**1.14**

polished rice, tea, salt, chocolate, and vegetable fats with a relatively smaller amount of milk, eggs, or meat. An example of the refined foods found in the modern Eskimo diet can be found on the next page.

Dr. Price explained that the modern diet is deficient in minerals compared to the traditional Eskimo diet (see traditional diet above):

> *Since their muscle meat, glands and other organs of animals of the land for the Indians and of the sea for the Eskimos, would be reduced approximately to one-tenth, this would decrease the total fat-soluble activators per day to* ***a quantity below the minimum bodily requirements of even an adult.*** *This will make it impossible for them to utilize properly even the small amount of minerals that are present in the foods ingested besides being insufficient to maintain the functioning of various organs and tissues of the body. It is at this point that their greatest injury occurs. Even if they could utilize all the minerals that are available the intake for those on modern foods is reduced to less than one fifth of that in the original diets for several of the minerals.*[26] *(Emphasis added.)*

Southern Pacific Islanders Experience Marked Gum Tissue Destruction

During the summer of 1934, Dr. Price visited the Southern Pacific Islands, including the Marquesas Islands, Society Island, Cook Island, Tongan Island, New Caledonia, Fiji Island, Samoan Islands, and the Hawaiian Islands.

South Sea Islanders living on their primitive native foods had healthy teeth, with only 0.34 percent of teeth attacked by tooth decay. In contrast, those eating the foods of modern civilization had cavities in 30.8 percent of their teeth.[27]

South Pacific Islanders ate liberal amounts of sea foods including organs and

The Beautiful Polynesians on Their Native Diets

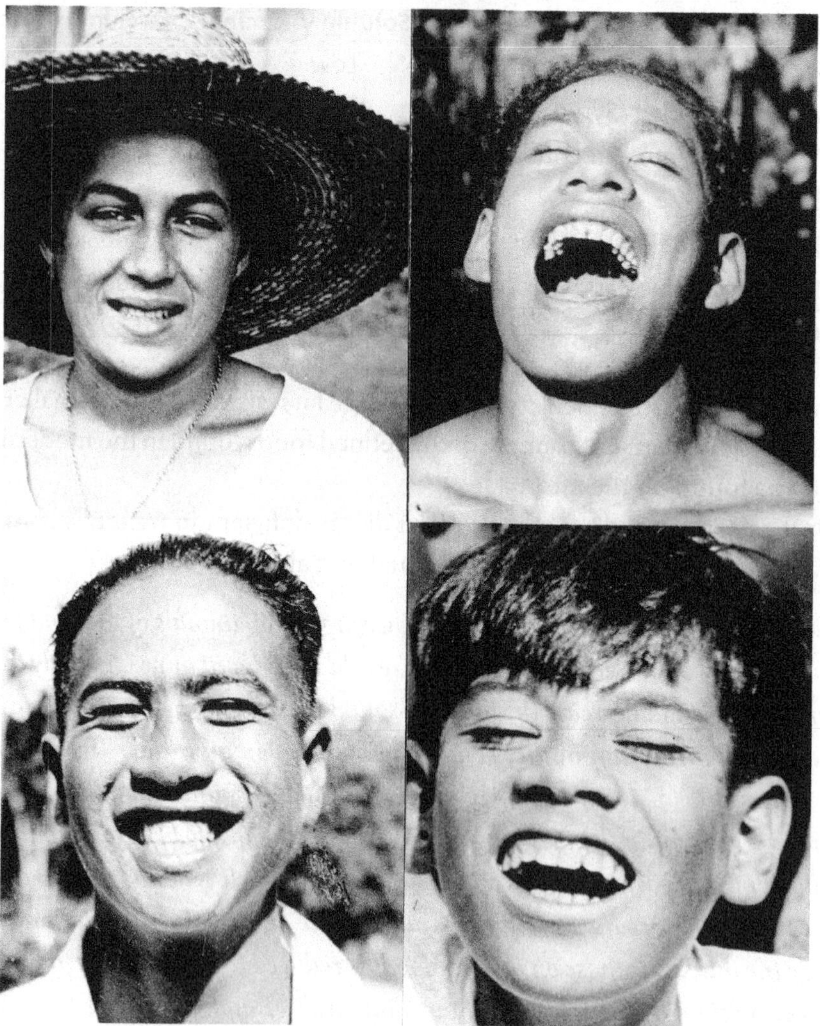

Polynesians are a beautiful race and physically sturdy. They have straight hair and their color is often that of a sun tanned European. They have perfect dental arches. (Original caption.)

eggs from sea animals, plus a wide variety of plant roots and fruits, both raw and cooked. The primary food eaten for carbohydrates was taro root; yams, sweet potatoes, and bread fruit were also eaten. Fruits such as bananas and papayas were consumed along with coconut. Sea life of every sort was consumed including crayfish, octopus, lobsters, oysters, clams, many types of large and small fish, as well as

When Polynesians Eat Modern Foods, Their Dental Health Deteriorates

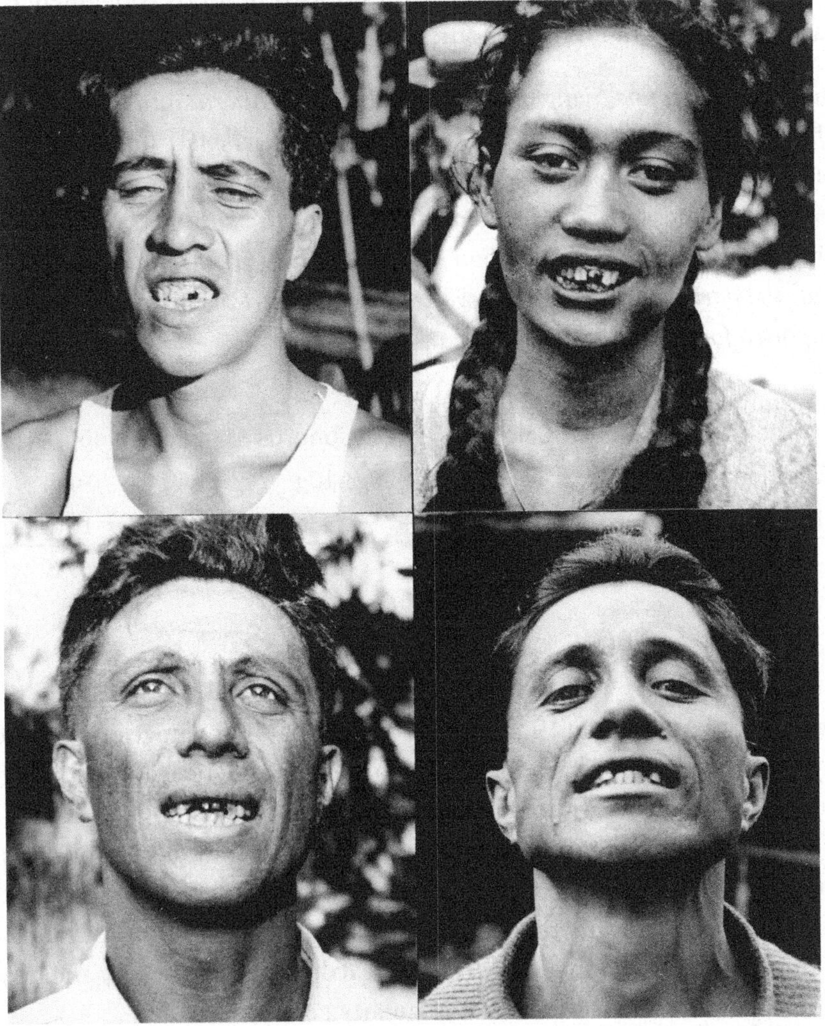

Wherever the native foods have been displaced by the imported foods, dental caries become rampant. These are typical modernized Tahitians. (Original caption.)

turtles. Fish head soup provided an abundance of minerals, and seaweed provided iodine. Even the eyes of the fish were eaten and valued for their nutrient content.[28]

Today South Pacific Islanders suffer from high rates of diabetes and obesity. Their diets are heavy in white flour, white sugar, canned meat and fish, margarine, mayonnaise, sodas, candies, cookies, and breakfast cereals.[29] Eight out of the ten most obese countries in the world are located in the South Pacific.[30]

Dr. Price noted how gum disease occurred when indigenous people who lived near the trading ports replaced their seafood with modern convenience foods—primarily white sugar and white flour.

> *In all of the groups living on native foods with a liberal intake of animal life of the sea, the health of the gums was generally excellent. When, however,* ***the sea foods were quite limited in the dietary,*** *heavy deposits formed and often were associated with a* ***marked destruction of the supporting tissues with gingival infection.*** *This condition was particularly prevalent among all groups near the ports, when the groups were displacing part of their native foods with imported foods.*[32] *(Emphasis added.)*

Diet Type	Calcium	Phosphorus	Fat-Soluble Vitamins
Traditional Diet[31]	1.9g	3.10g	High
Processed Diet	0.97g	1.36g	Low
Difference	*53%*	*56%*	*67%*

The Message of the Aborigines of Australia

Dr. Price visited Australia in 1936. He discovered that the average rate of tooth decay among Australia's native Aborigines was zero percent, which means that they had total immunity to tooth decay. In contrast, he found that the average decay rate of all teeth of modern Aborigines living on reservations and eating modern foods was 71 percent of all teeth.[33]

Dr. Price observed that the Australian Aborigines, who for thousands of years maintained near-perfect physical forms, have lost their ideal beauty and health with the foods that our modern society so regularly consumes.

Traditional Diet of Native Aborigines

The Aboriginal diet was a hunter-gatherer diet.

> *For plant foods they used roots, stems, leaves, berries and seeds of grasses and a native pea eaten with tissues of large and small animals. The large animals available are the kangaroo and wallaby. Among the small animals they have a variety of rodents, insects, beetles and grubs, and wherever available various forms of animal life from the rivers and oceans. Birds and birds' eggs are used where available.*[35]

Aborigines of Australia

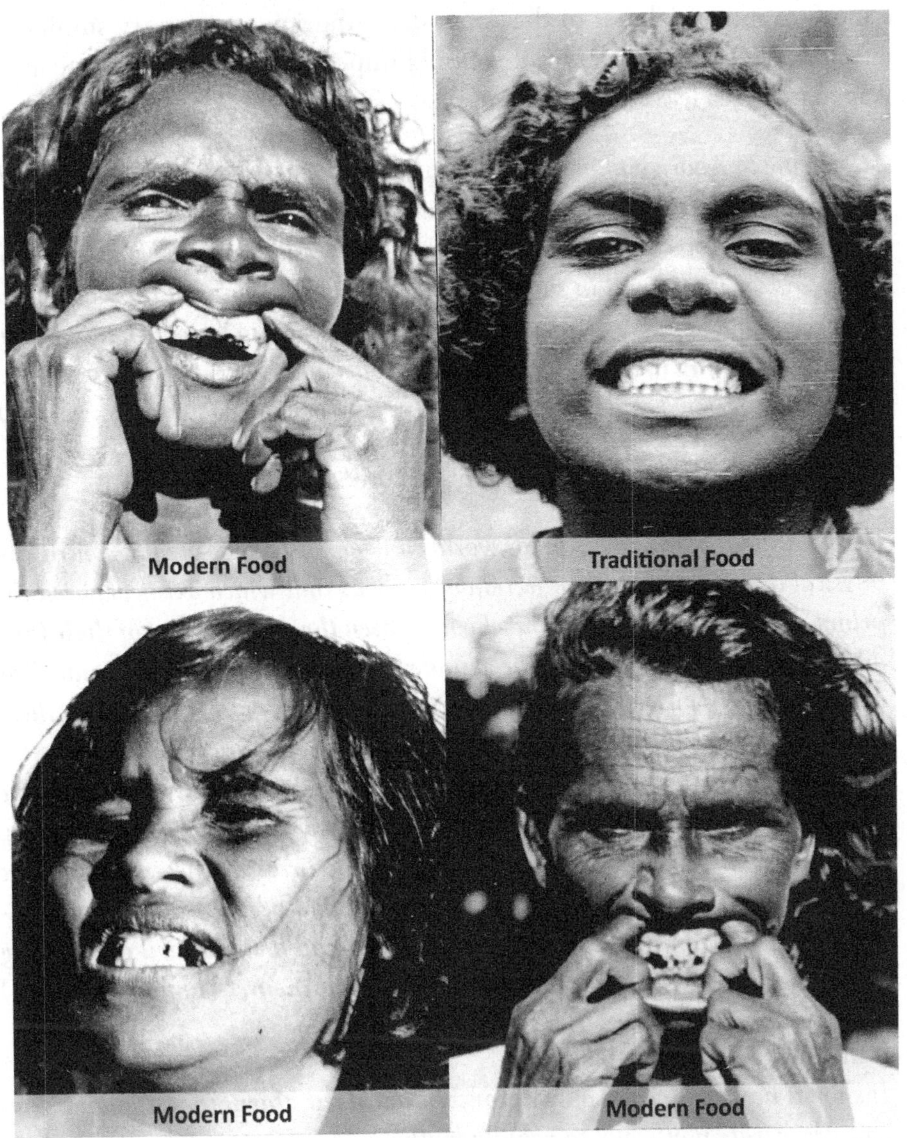

Wherever the primitive Aborigines have been placed in reservations and fed on the white man's foods of commerce dental caries has become rampant. This destroys their beauty, prevents mastication, and provides infection for seriously injuring their bodies. Note the contrast between the primitive woman in the upper right and the three modernized women.[34] (Original caption.)

Modern Industrial Aboriginal Diet That Created Poor Oral Health

The modern industrial diet of the Australian Aborigines was very similar to the other modernized diets listed in this book. Imported foods included sugar, flour, packaged milk, tea leaves, and meat in tins.[36]

> *[Referring to Aboriginal picture on the previous page:] Note the contrast with the upper right. It is quite impossible to imagine the suffering that these people were compelled to endure due to abscessing teeth resulting from rampant tooth decay. As we had found in some of the modernized islands of the Pacific, we discovered that here, too,* ***discouragement and a longing for death had taken the place of a joy in living in many****. Few souls in the world have experienced this discouragement and this longing to a greater degree.* [37] *(Emphasis added.)*

His poetic words paint an important picture:

> *It is doubtful if many places in the world can demonstrate so great a contrast in physical development and perfection of body as that which exists between the primitive Aborigines of Australia who have been* ***the sole arbiters of their fate****, and those Aborigines who have been under the influence of the white man. The white man has deprived them of their original habitats and is now feeding them in reservations while using them as laborers in modern industrial pursuits.*
>
> *I have seldom, if ever, found* ***whites suffering so tragically*** *from evidence of physical degeneration, as expressed in tooth decay and change in facial form, as are the whites of eastern Australia. This has occurred on the very best of the land that these [aboriginals] formerly occupied and becomes at once a monument to the wisdom of the primitive Aborigines and* ***a signboard of warning to the modern civilization that has supplanted them****.*[38] *(Emphasis added.)*

A dire warning from Dr. Price:

> *It should be a matter not only of concern but* ***deep alarm*** *that human beings can degenerate physically so rapidly by the use of a certain type of nutrition, particularly the dietary products used so generally by modern civilization.*[39] *(Emphasis added.)*

Nutritive Values of Diets Compared

Weston Price performed nutrient analyses of the foods eaten by many of the isolated and modernized groups he studied. He consistently found dramatic differences when he compared the nutritional content of the native diets to their modern replacements. On average, the ancestral diet had two to four times more copper, magnesium, iron, calcium, phosphorous, iodine, and other minerals; and at least ten times the fat soluble vitamins A, D, E, and K.[40] This data is visualized in the following chart:

The Dramatic Difference in Dietary Nutrients Discovered by Dr. Price.

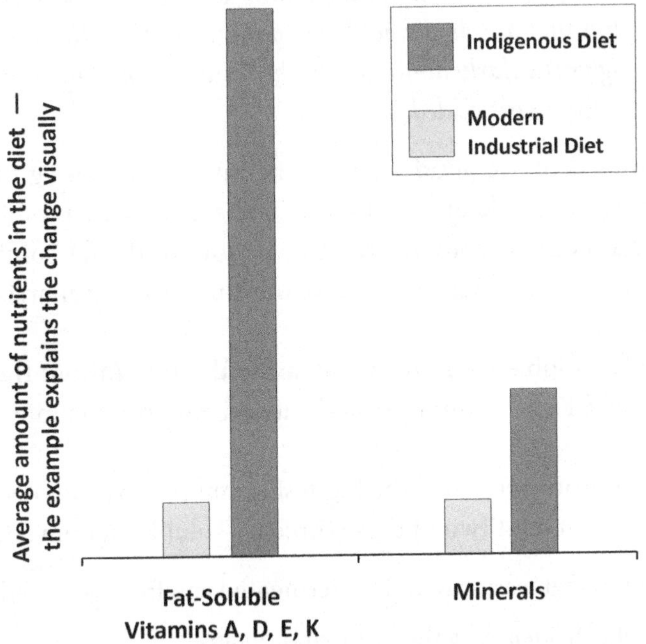

Dr. Price had little doubt that the nutrient-poor industrial diet caused gum disease in modern civilization. He attributed loss of bone, including loss of the periodontium, to the body's need to steal needed minerals for use in other bodily tissues and organs.

> *We have many other expressions of this borrowing process. Much of what we have thought of as so-called pyorrhea in which the bone is progressively lost from around the teeth thus allowing them to loosen, constitutes one of the most common phases of the borrowing process. This tissue with its lowered defense rapidly becomes infected and we think of the process largely in terms of that infection. A part of the local process includes the deposit of so-called calculus and tartar about the teeth. These contain toxic substances which greatly irritate the flesh starting an inflammatory reaction.* ***Pyorrhea in the light of our newer knowledge is largely a nutritional problem.***[41] *(Emphasis added.)*

Fat-soluble Vitamins and Activators: A Secret to Gum Disease Reversal

Dr. Price wrote that gum disease (pyorrhea) is a problem of a lack of nutrients in our diet.

> *Nutrition plus the frequent removal of deposits, plus suitable medication will* ***check and prevent pyorrhea*** *but not correct the damage that has already been done. The elements that are chiefly needed in our nutrition are those that I have outlined as being particularly abundant in the menus as used by several of the primitive races. (Emphasis added.)*

His advice to us is to use good nutrition and manual cleaning of calculus to prevent gum disease and to keep the disease in check. And as a reminder, "good nutrition" means a diet that contains ten times more of the fat-soluble vitamins than we have in our modern diet, and two to four times more minerals than in our normal diet.

To get those fat-soluble vitamins, **think animal fats**. Without the fat-soluble vitamins A, D, E, and K, we cannot properly absorb and use the minerals present in our diets.

The indigenous groups that had the highest immunity to tooth decay and gum disease ate daily from at least two of these three fat-soluble vitamin sources:

- ☐ Dairy products that were raw and/or fermented and from grass-fed animals.
- ☐ Fish and shellfish, including the heads and organs.
- ☐ Organs of land animals.

In a forgotten 1936 article from the *Journal of the American Dental Association*, Dr. Price revealed a little known secret for 100 percent immunity from tooth decay and gum disease:

> *On the basis of the fat-soluble activators or vitamin content of the foods used, I found that those groups using at least two of the three* ***principal vitamin sources*** *had the highest immunity to dental caries. Those using the lowest amount of fat-soluble activators had the greatest amount of dental caries. On this basis, namely, the fat-soluble activator content of the diet, those groups using the fat-soluble activators in liberal quantity had not more than 0.5 per cent of the teeth attacked by dental caries; while those using fat-soluble activators less liberally had up to 12 per cent of the teeth attacked by dental caries.* ***All groups having a liberal supply of minerals*** *particularly phosphorus, and* ***a liberal supply of fat-soluble activators****, had* ***100 per cent immunity*** *to dental caries.*[42] *(Emphasis added.)*

The remedy for gum disease, since the condition is opposite in some ways to tooth decay, is slightly different—it's plenty of minerals including **calcium** with **fat-soluble vitamins** from the organs of land and/or sea animals, along with excellent grass-fed dairy products that will produce immunity and remission of gum disease.

Vegans do not any eat animal products and vegetarians often do not consume plenty of dairy products. This means many of them suffer from deficiencies of calcium, phosphorus, and fat-soluble vitamins. For example, it's unfortunately a myth that most people can convert beta carotene into fat-soluble vitamin A. Rates of conversion vary from modest to not at all, and even when conversion is possible, many more units of beta carotene are necessary to produce only small units of true vitamin A. Children do not make the conversion at all.

Yes, it is possible to produce vitamin D in our skin from exposure to the sun. But it hard but it is hard to produce optimal amounts when living far from the equator even while being naked out in the sun most of the day, and even if being naked in the sun sounds like fun to you!

Vitamin K1 from plant foods is not going to give the same result in preventing gum disease as vitamin K2 from animal foods. The lack of true fat-soluble vitamins and calcium in the vegan diet makes it difficult for vegans over time to remain immune to tooth decay or gum disease, which are effects of physical degeneration. Vegetarians who are committed to finding top-quality foods can do okay, but have a much harder time because of the limited food selection and lack of food sources for the B vitamins and vitamin D.

What Other Foods Might Help?

Eggs can be an excellent source of fat-soluble vitamins, but only if sourced from pastured hens that primarily eat insects, and not too many grains. Store-bought eggs from chickens fed on corn and soy, even if organic and non-GMO, lack the high level of vitamins and other nutrients we need to prevent and reverse gum disease.

Insects

Those of us who can get past the "yuck" factor will find insects to be an excellent source of minerals, protein, and they have a nice crunch too! My children actually love eating grasshoppers. Fatty insects will likely be rich in fat-soluble vitamins that are missing in our modern industrial diet.

To summarize, our modern diet rarely includes the traditional foods that isolated indigenous people ate, which made them immune to both tooth decay and gum disease. Do you eat fish with the heads? How about liver, bone marrow, heart, or blood curd? While Americans do favor dairy products, most are of inferior quality and commercial dairy products can make people sick due to confinement animal feeding operations producing inferior milk, not to mention the fact that most milk sold in America is pasteurized, or even ultra pasteurized and homogenized, which diminishes the nutrient content and renders the milk toxic.

Why Do We Have Gum Disease in Modern Civilization?

The short answer is we do not eat the same food that our ancestors ate and we fail to get enough of the vitamins and minerals that our body needs. The result for far too many people today is bone loss in the jaw (gum disease).

A typical adult needs to eat approximately the following nutrients, daily, to be healthy:

Nutritional Guidelines Based on Weston Price's Research

Calcium	Phosphorus	Vitamin A	Vitamin D	Percent of Calories from Fat
1.5 grams	2 grams	4,000 – 20,000 IU	1,000 – 4,000 IU	25-65+%

What about Synthetic Vitamins?

Synthetic vitamins can help sometimes, but they are not usually effective in the long run and they usually have unintended side effects because their actions in the body are so specific

The figures for calcium and phosphorus come from Dr. Price himself. The figures for the vitamins A and D and the calories from fat are based on my analysis of several different interpretations of healthy diets as well as recommendations from the Weston A. Price Foundation, www.westonaprice.org. These figures are general guidelines and may not be suited for all readers. You will need to modify these guidelines depending on your level of health, your weight, and your dietary needs.

The U.S. Government also has dietary standards, called the DRI, Dietary Reference Intake, formerly called the RDA, Recommended Dietary Allowances. These standards are far lower than the vitamin and nutritional standards of healthy indigenous groups around the globe. Even with these much lower standards, many people today do not meet the requirements. For example, on average 65 percent of the population is deficient in calcium, 54 percent deficient in vitamin B6, 56 percent of the population is deficient in vitamin A, and 73 percent of the population deficient in zinc.[43]

It isn't a mystery why nearly half of the adult population has some gum recession, and 38.5 percent has moderate or severe periodontal disease? Clearly, even by the U.S. Government data the average person does not get enough vitamins and minerals to be healthy. This is because consuming our modern refined diet makes it very difficult for us to meet our bodies' minimum standard requirements for nutrient intakes.

To connect our discussion back to the first chapter of this book, I gave you evidence of how the dental profession has focused on bacteria and ignored the idea of host response. Now we can see in this chapter that the modern food we eat affects whether we get tooth decay or gum disease. In general tooth decay and gum disease are the most visible signs of nutrient depletion. By ignoring how nutrition affects our bodies and by blaming bacteria for dental health problems, the field of dentistry does us a great disservice by diverting us from the truth of how a poor diet causes gum disease and tooth decay.

The Forgotten Spirit of Service

In the spirit of ancestral wisdom that we as a culture do not revere, I'd like to cite Dr. Price's comments about the original people of Australia. He wrote:

> *The boys and girls are taught the names of the great characters that make up the different constellations.* ***These were individuals who had conquered all of the temptations of life*** *and had lived so* ***completely in the interest of others*** *that they had fulfilled the great motivating principle of their religion, which is* ***that life consists in serving others as one would wish to be served****. (Emphasis added.)*

The concept of living in service to others is not unique to the Aboriginal people; it is found in many great religions and cultures.

In general our modern society is not built upon the spirit of service, but upon the spirit of material gain, and upon exploiting nature. If we are to measure the results of our civilization by its actions, such as the ability to treat chronic disease like gum disease, we can see that it is failing. We have a dental industry in which many, although not all, dentists have lost their way. There is a focus on making the most profit rather than on providing selfless service to patients who are suffering. While our society continues to crumble around us as it must, I invite you to remember the spirit of the great religions of the world: do good to others, and likewise, do good for yourself.

3 Know the True Nature of the Cause of Gum Disease

Modern dentistry does not offer nutritionally based preventative or adjunct treatments. Its treatment methods are based on the bacterial theory which modern science has shown is not accurate. Allow me to introduce you to two pioneers in the dental health profession who looked at the etiology of gum disease holistically. What they have found has dramatic implications for the future of dentistry.

The Work of Dentist Harold Hawkins

One such extraordinary dentist was Dr. Harold F. Hawkins, a noted dental surgeon and a former associate professor at the University of Southern California. He had a strong interest in nutrition and was a follower of the work of Dr. Weston Price.

Over the course of twenty years, Dr. Hawkins studied more than eight thousand individual cases of dental health problems with scientific precision, and reported his research in the groundbreaking book *Applied Nutrition* published in 1940. Just as the more recent dental literature has established today, Dr. Hawkins knew more than seventy years ago that "a very sizable percentage of [gum disease] cases [are] purely metabolic in character and in these cases bacteria and tissue pockets play absolutely no part."[1]

Like many dentists in practice prior to World War II, Dr. Hawkins saw his role as more than a cosmetic filler of teeth. He recognized that the beginnings of imbalances in health and chronic disease were visible in the mouth and considered it his duty to try to stop gum disease and tooth loss at the level of causation. To this end he avidly studied body chemistry, experimented in the laboratory, applied his findings to his patients, and reported his outcomes in his writings.

Gum Health according to Dr. Hawkins

Dr. Hawkins believed that healthy tissues in the mouth are a result of cells throughout the body being adequately nourished with all necessary vitamins, minerals, and hormones. Any disturbance in the free flow of nourishment and in the removal of waste products at the cellular level can cause gum recession. He also noted that abnormal stress on the teeth and biting forces can degrade gum health.[2]

Dr. Hawkins believed the following conditions must be met in order to ensure for healthy oral tissues:

- There must be adequate minerals, vitamins, and hormones from an optimum, well-balanced diet.
- The mouth and blood pH must be balanced, with good circulation down to the cellular level so that cellular waste products are released from the body.
- The gums require stimulation via the massaging action of the chewing process.
- If there are dental restorations, they must not inflame gum tissue or cause bite problems because they are too high or too low.
- The entire body must be restored to good health.
- There must be plenty of saliva flow to protect and mineralize the gums and teeth.

Healthy Gums Are Fed by Nutrient-Rich Body Fluids

The alveolar bone is the ridge of bone (jawbone) that contains the sockets of the teeth and supports the teeth. In dry form it is composed of 67 percent calcium phosphate, a combination of calcium and phosphorous arranged in a formation called hydroxyapatite, with a smaller percentage of trace minerals, 28 percent of mostly type 1 collagen, and 5 percent proteins.[3] Alveolar bone contains about 15 percent fluid, and receives its blood supply through the main arteries of the maxilla

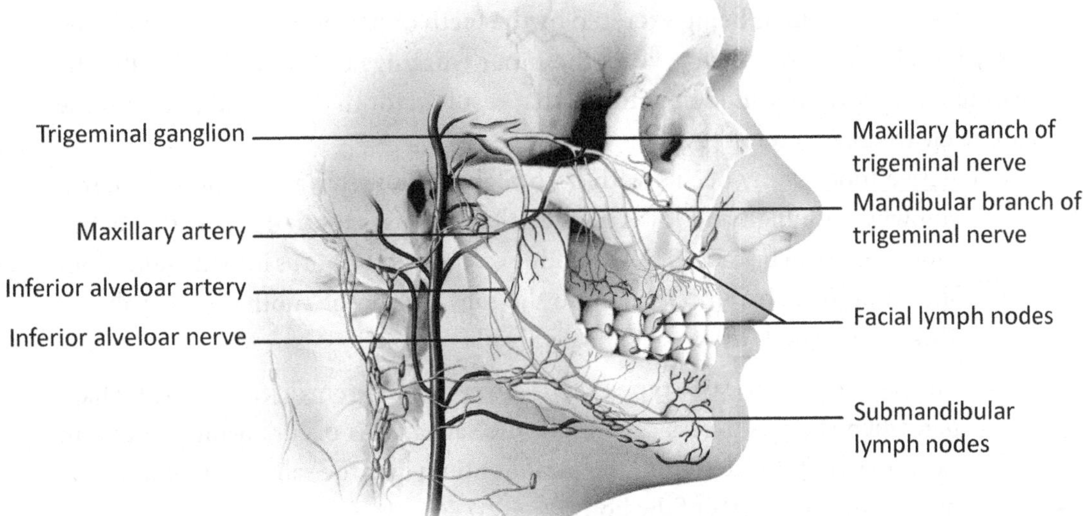

and mandible. The bone is also supplied with submandibular lymph nodes and fluid, as well as branches of nerves.

The nourishment to the gum tissue, ligaments, nerves, and alveolar bone is supplied through the circulatory and fluid system. As people suffer from physical deterioration, the vital nutrient supply to the periodontium becomes critically restricted and cellular regeneration slows. As a result, when people lose their health with age and subsequently lose their teeth from gum disease, they are actually suffering from **profound bone loss** throughout their body. The place where bone loss is most visible for many people is in the alveolar bone.

Hawkins' pH and Calcium Measurements

Dr. Hawkins measured the saliva, blood, and urine concentrations of calcium and phosphorous in various states of periodontal health and disease. He found distinct imbalances in the bone-building minerals calcium and phosphorous in people with tooth decay and gum disease.

This valuable chart summarizes the body chemistry patterns from tests of hundreds of individuals. The horizontal line shows the saliva buffer pH. For our purposes, think that anything less than the ideal mark represents that the saliva, and therefore the body has become more acidic than is ideal for optimal health. The vertical line shows the milligrams of calcium per cubic centimeter (denoted as cc, 5 cc = 1 teaspoon) of saliva. Again, for our purposes the exact figures are not as important as the overall picture that Dr. Hawkins' research revealed. In the chart, low salivary calcium (toward the top of the chart) usually indicates calcium is being utilized by the body, and high salivary calcium (toward the bottom of the chart) indicates that calcium is being excreted by the teeth or periodontium. Reproduced here, Dr. Hawkins' research reveals the inner workings of the body. Finally, the distinct and previously hidden patterns that result in tooth decay and gum disease can be clearly seen. Here they are:

- Active tooth decay occurs with both high and low salivary calcium. The reason why both high and low salivary calcium causes tooth decay is that active tooth decay can be caused by the body excreting phosphorus into the saliva (not shown on this chart), calcium into the saliva, or both. Tooth decay is almost always associated with an acidic salivary pH.
- Both active gum disease (type I) and slower wasting gum disease (type II) happen when there is excess calcium in the saliva. This occurs primarily due to calcium being chelated from the periodontium into the saliva so that it can be utilized by other parts of the body.

Tooth Decay and Gum Disease in Relationship to Saliva Buffer pH and Salivary Calcium

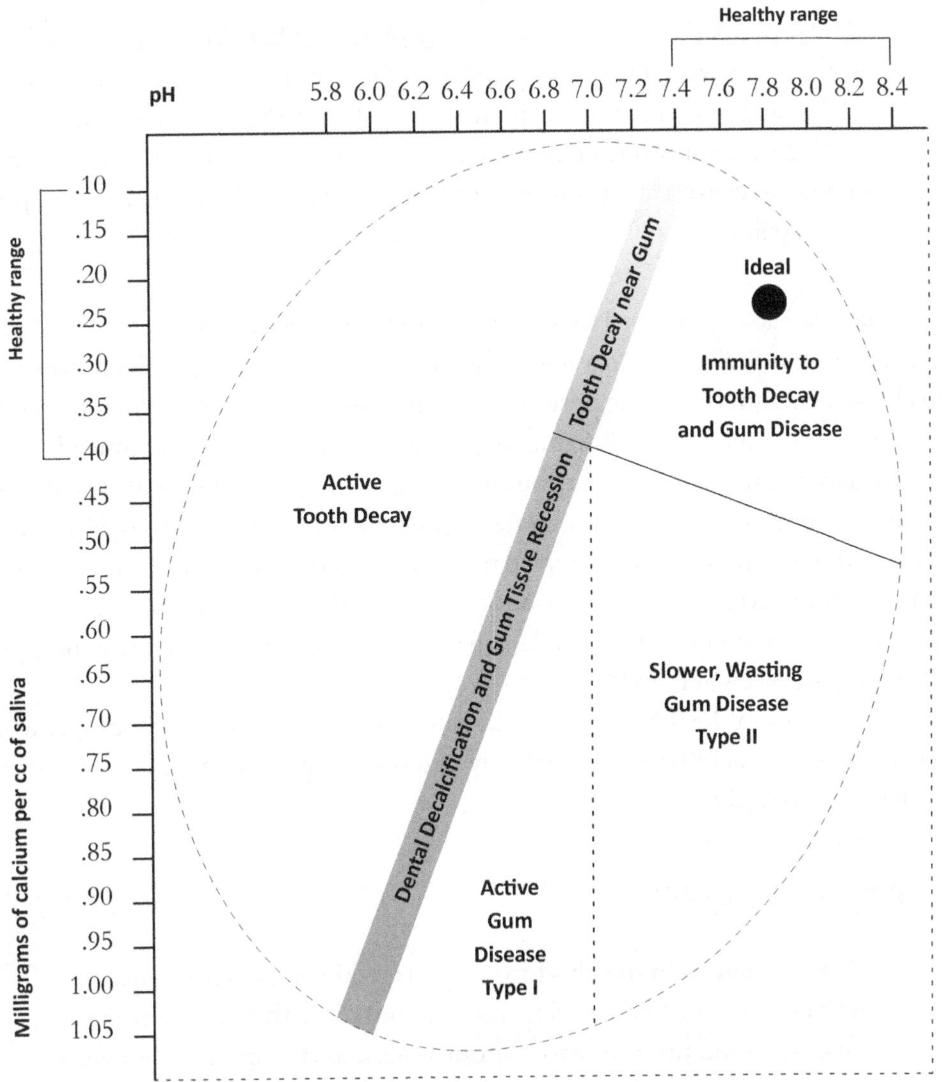

- ☐ With severe gum disease the salivary pH is acidic; this generally indicates deeper imbalances in the body, poor digestion, and a lack of fat-soluble vitamins.
- ☐ <u>Immunity to tooth decay and gum disease</u> happens when the body is utilizing both calcium and phosphorous and when the body is not excreting those minerals into the saliva due to adequate calcium and phosphorous intake and utilization. The *ideal* point on the chart shows that when the salivary pH is balanced, tooth decay does not occur.

- Tooth decay near the gum line occurs when there is some acidity and some phosphorous loss, but the loss is not as severe as what would cause cavities on the crowns (tops) of the teeth.
- Dental decalcification and gum tissue recession happens to people who fall in a zone between tooth decay and gum disease. Their body is acidic and they are loosing calcium and phosphorous, but it is neither severe enough to cause tooth decay, nor severe enough to cause significant gum disease. But it is severe enough to cause a loss of enamel, and sensitive gum tissues which will be prone to recession.

The more acidic saliva pH associated with tooth decay and severe gum disease occurs because the body is in a state of acidosis. In this state, it is easier for the body to chelate calcium out of the periodontium to more vital organs. When the body's chemistry is in balance and inflammation is low, calcium loss is minimized.[4]

In many cases of severe periodontal disease, large amounts of calculus and plaque are present as calcium migrates out of the teeth or jaw bones and into the saliva.[5] This is what Dr. Price referred to as the "borrowing process," in which minerals are transferred from the periodontium to other tissues and organs. In plain language, when minerals are pulled from teeth or bones, they do not just disappear. They migrate elsewhere in the body.

To regain oral health, people need to move back into the ideal range, which means removing acidity from their body and restoring calcium and other minerals back into their body.

pH and Oral Health

The pH figures in the chart from Dr. Hawkins represent buffer pH values. The salivary samples were in contact with the colorimetric hydrogen-ion test indicator for one hour and the pH test was taken in between meals. Dr. Hawkins believed this test showed the buffering ability of saliva. The pH figures in the chart are not meant to be used as a one-to-one reference with pH paper readings.

You can test your urinary and saliva pH at home with pH paper or strips. But the ideal salivary and urine pH is 6.4 according to RBTI (Reams Biological Theory of Ionization). Any reading above or below 6.4 indicates your body is out of balance.

Relationship of Calcium and Phosphorus to Tooth Decay and Gum Disease

Tooth Decay

	Calcium	Phosphorous
Saliva	Low	High
Blood	High	Low
Urine	High	Low

Gum Disease

	Calcium	Phosphorous
Saliva	High	Low
Blood	Low	High
Urine	Low	High

The cause of gum disease according to Dr. Hawkins is the loss of calcium that is systemic in nature:

> *In gum disease, the body is not able to hold its calcium or the intake does not balance the loss. As a result there is a disintegration of the alveolar process surrounding the teeth and the eventual loss of teeth.* **All other bones of the body are affected** *but because the alveolar bone is quite spongy in character the loss is more apparent than in the denser bones of the body.*[6] *(Emphasis added.)*

A recent study has confirmed some of Dr. Hawkins' research showing that high salivary calcium is related to periodontal disease.[7]

Dr. Hawkins discovered three distinct patterns for gum disease.

Type 1 Gum Disease	High Calculus Deposits	75% of Cases

- ☐ Low blood levels of calcium with high blood levels of phosphorous.
- ☐ Inflamed gums with tissue pockets and general gum bleeding.
- ☐ Loss of density and flattening of the alveolar process due to bone destruction.
- ☐ Alkalinity of saliva is depressed resulting in acidic saliva.[8]

Dr. Hawkins reported that this is the most prevalent form of gum disease, appearing in 75 percent of cases. It shows itself in blood chemistry as low blood calcium along with high blood phosphorous. This happens because calcium is being pulled out of the body. The result is a relatively elevated level of phosphorous as well as acidic saliva. When the relationship between calcium and phosphorous in the body is disturbed, gum disease will result.[9]

In addition to calcium and phosphorous, Dr. Hawkins believed that vitamins A, B, and C were very important to resolving this condition. Dr. Hawkins also notes that in instances of advanced infection in the gum tissues, it is difficult for the infected tissue to regenerate without the infected area being cleared up with manual interventions.

Dr. Hawkins found that Type 1 gum disease was sometimes associated with a diet high in potassium and fat, as well as in conditions of poor salt retention (see chapter six for list of high potassium high fat foods to avoid). The specifics of this condition, while not described, point out some things to be aware of in relation to gum disease:

1. Eating modern industrial vegetable fats (a full list is in chapter six) can cause or contribute to gum disease.
2. Eating healthy fats when the liver is not able to metabolize them correctly can contribute to gum disease.
3. Dr. Price found both fat-soluble vitamins and minerals are deficient in our modern diet. Increasing fat-soluble vitamin intake without increasing mineral intake could lead to mineral deficiencies because natural animal fats need "mineral friends" with which to work together to build bone density and create metabolic harmony.

Therefore, people consuming high fat diets who have gum disease need to examine a few possibilities. One is that it is possible that the fat is not being properly metabolized. Another is that people **who eat more fat need to also consume plenty of trace minerals**, from organic kelp (and other seafood), as well as dietary calcium.

Type 2 Gum Disease	No Calculus Deposits	23% of Cases

- ☐ Blood levels of both calcium and phosphorus are low.
- ☐ The gum tone is good and there is generally no bleeding on probing.
- ☐ Gums not usually receded yet there is a general wasting and destruction of the alveolar process.
- ☐ Teeth tend to be loose.
- ☐ Absence of calculus deposits (hardened dental plaque).

This type of gum disease is found in 23 percent of cases and is caused by significant mineral deficiencies. Due to low levels of phosphorous, calcium is not properly mobilized and it is being excreted into the saliva. In Type 2 gum disease, the body uses up more calcium and phosphorous than is being taken in by the diet. This type of gum disease has no pocket formations or infections. It is caused by a deficiency of calcium, phosphorous, and the activating fat-soluble vitamins, A, D, E, and K. This type is much easier to resolve than Type 1 because it indicates that the main disturbance is a deficiency condition.[10] In comparison, Type 1 gum disease presents more serious underlying imbalances resulting in more severe symptoms.

Type 3 Gum Disease	Abundant Calculus Deposits	2% of Cases

- Blood levels of calcium are high while blood levels of phosphorous are low.
- Good gum tone with minor irritations.
- Evidence of both alveolar bone loss and flattening.
- Abundant calculus deposits.

This is the least common type of gum disease and is generally accompanied by tooth decay. Dr. Hawkins blamed the disturbed calcium metabolism on "aggravating factors of body chemistry," which could include excessive internal magnesium or sulphur, drugs or medications that block calcium metabolism, low stomach acid, poor thyroid function,[11] mercury poisoning, mold, and galvanic currents.

Gum Disease	Type 1-75% of cases	Type 2-23% of cases	Type 3-2% of cases
Blood Calcium Levels	Low	Low	High
Blood Phosphorus Levels	High	Low	Low
Gum Condition	Inflamed, tissue pockets, bleeding	Good, no bleeding on probing, generally not receding	Good gum tone with minor irritations
Alveolar Process	Loss of density and flattening	General wasting and destruction	Evidence of both alveolar bone loss and flattening
Teeth	Erosion or normal	Loose	Generally accompanied by decay
Saliva	Acidic	Neutral	N/a
Calculus Deposits	Above and below gums	Absent	Abundant

Dentist Melvin Page's Good Chemistry

Dentist Melvin Page (1894 –1983) began to make his mark in the dental field by developing dentures that fit better than those typical of his day. As a prosthodontist, he noticed a serious problem: even patients without teeth needed new dentures within two and a half years because their jaw bones would resorb (deteriorate) even more, causing their dentures not to fit! While investigating the cause of periodontal bone loss that progressed even in people without teeth or gum pockets,

The Biochemical Cause of Gum Disease and Tooth Decay

After thirty years and forty thousand blood tests, Dr. Page discovered and confirmed the biochemical conditions that cause tooth decay and gum disease: a disturbance in the ratio of calcium to phosphorus in the blood. A ratio of 8.75mg of calcium per 100cc of blood, and 3.5mg of phosphorus per 100cc of blood, with normal blood sugar levels, creates immunity to both tooth decay and gum disease.[13] The healthy blood sugar level is around 85 milligrams per 100 cc of blood.[14] If those two criteria are met, then alveolar bone resorption ceases.

Dr. Page found the work of Dr. Price.[12]

When there is a low level of blood phosphorus over a period of several months then tooth decay develops.[15] And based on this same research, **when there is a low level of blood calcium over a period of months, gum disease begins.**

A Real Cause of Calculus

Dr. Page thought calculus deposits above the gum line indicated a high blood calcium level in relation to the amount of phosphorous present. Conversely, as Dr. Hawkins found, irritated gums and calculus below the gum line toward the root of the tooth occurred when blood phosphorus becomes too high in relationship to blood calcium (in other words, the blood calcium is too low).

A Real Cause of Gingivitis

Dr. Page reported that gingivitis was caused by a low calcium and high phosphorus ratio. He wrote that the blood could often be "cleared up without surgical interference" by reducing the phosphorous level to the correct proportions.[16]

Based on Dr. Page's model, gingivitis can be a precursor to periodontal disease not because of bacteria, but because of the related, although less severe, imbalance in the blood chemistry.

To summarize, the method Dr. Page and Dr. Hawkins used to heal gum disease was to create balance between the calcium and phosphorous ratios in the blood. This was achieved with a combination of dietary interventions, supplements and glandular concentrates. In the most common type of gum disease, which Dr. Hawkins called Type 1, the blood calcium is too low relative to blood phosphorous. In Type 2 gum disease, both the blood calcium and blood phosphorous are low. Both of these conditions are the result of significant vitamin and mineral deficiencies.

Our Neuroendocrine System and Gum Disease

Dr. Page found that our autonomic (automatic) nervous system and our endocrine (glandular/hormonal) system are directly affected by the food we eat. Because of the close relationship between these two systems, they can be referred to together as the neuroendocrine system. Every function in our body is orchestrated by our neuroendocrine system. The nervous system and the endocrine (glandular) system are linked together in the hypothalamus of our brain by the pituitary gland. When the hypothalamus detects changes in the body, it sends messages to the pituitary gland and to our autonomic nervous system to tell them how to function and respond to the situation.[17]

In states of disease, Dr. Page found that these two systems become disregulated. It turns out that when our calcium and phosphorus levels are out of balance in our blood, so too are the autonomic nervous system and endocrine system out of balance.

Our autonomic nervous system controls the involuntary processes of our organs and glands such as heart rate, digestion, respiratory rate, salivation, perspiration, urination, sexual arousal, breathing, and swallowing. Our autonomic system has three divisions: enteric, parasympathic, and sympathetic. The enteric system, which governs the gastrointestinal system, is left out of this discussion, yet it may be worth further investigation.

The **sympathetic system** promotes the "fight or flight" response and is the speed up system. It corresponds with arousal and energy and it inhibits digestion by pulling blood away from the digestive tract and diverting it to large muscles. If **blood phosphorus is high** (usually with gum disease), the individual is overly using the sympathetic (active) nervous system and/or suppressing the parasympathetic (resting) system.

The **parasympathetic system** promotes the "rest and digest" response. It helps calm the nerves and slow the body down for digestion and resting. If **blood calcium is high** (most often found with tooth decay), the individual is overly in the parasympathetic state, so they are resting and going slow, and suppressing the sympathetic (speed up) system.

In the majority of cases of gum disease, the blood phosphorus is high, which means that the sympathetic nervous system is overactive, and/or the parasympathetic nervous system is suppressed. Some of the other illnesses that follow this pattern are arthritis, cancer, and diabetes.[18]

In general, people with gum disease have problems resting, digesting, and slowing down, and have a tendency towards emotional irritability. Healthy people constantly use both their active and the relaxing systems as the nervous system is meant to fluctuate throughout the day and even moment to moment, emphasizing one nervous system pathway over the other depending on the situation. Understanding the habitual nervous system dysfunction associated with gum disease gives us insight on how to treat the condition from a variety of perspectives. In particular it helps us hone in on the fact that people with gum disease need to improve their digestion. I will discuss ways to improve digestion in the discussion on diet in chapter eight. It also may indicate that people with gum disease may benefit from finding ways to manage and reduce stress.

Our Glandular System and Gum Disease

Gum disease is a whole body imbalance and not just an isolated oral problem. Dr. Page observed that out-of-balance calcium and phosphorous ratios could be brought into balance by correcting the functioning of the glandular system.[19] He also found that one of the chief functions of the glandular system was to support the digestive and metabolic processes.[20] When our glands are not working well, we will not metabolize food well.

Each gland in our body—with the exception of our adrenal glands—has both sympathetic and parasympathetic nerve wiring and functions. In contrast, the adrenal glands are only wired to the sympathetic (speed up) system.

Our endocrine system is composed of the pineal gland, pituitary gland, hypothalamus, thyroid, thymus, parathyroid, adrenal glands, pancreas, and ovaries or testes. These non-glandular organs also produce hormones: heart, kidney, digestive tract, and fat.[21] When we consume hormone-secreting glands and organs from healthy animals, we can help balance our body chemistry by giving nourishment

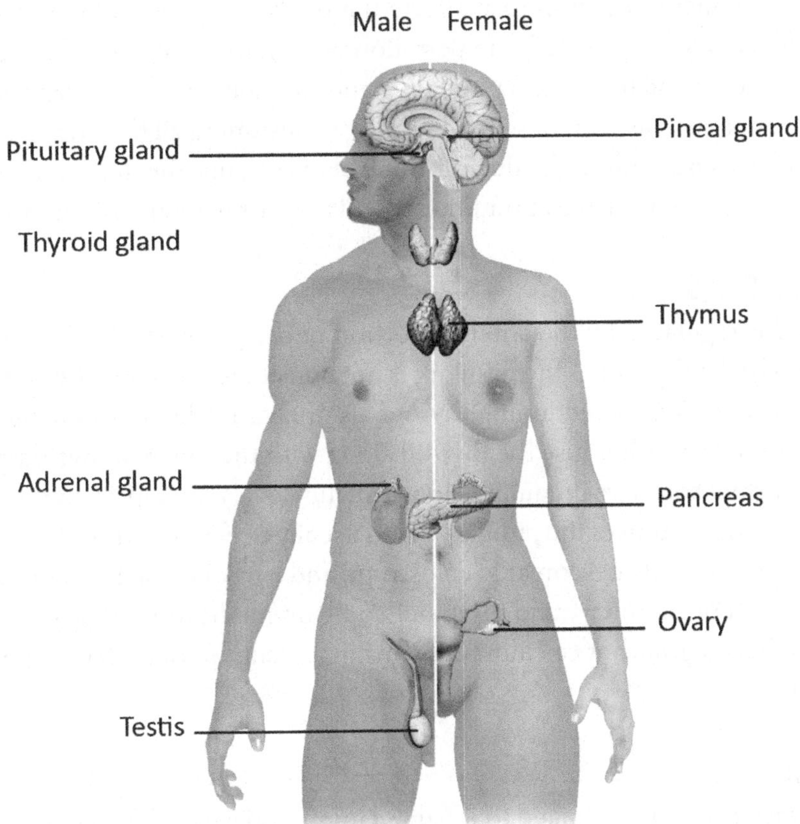

Our glands are the arbitrators of the major functions of our body.

to our glands. Perhaps that is why indigenous cultures found the organs and glands in the animals they hunted to be both vital and essential to their health. Two of the three sacred food categories that Dr. Price found that produce a high level of health and oral health, good bone structure, and immunity to disease are the organs and glands of land and sea animals.

Our individually inherited tendencies that determine our glandular strengths or weaknesses are likely what predispose some of us, when deficient in minerals and overall nutrition, to suffer from tooth decay, while others, with the same deficiency, suffer from gum disease.

The Pituitary Gland

Dr. Page noted that many cases of severe periodontal disease are associated with a deficiency in the posterior portion of the pituitary gland. The posterior part of the pituitary does not primarily affect blood sugar, but it does affect the calcium/phosphorous metabolism, which in turn affects the teeth and gums. When posterior pituitary deficiency is corrected, the periodontal condition improves.[22] The pituitary gland is corrected by taking a pituitary gland supplement, or by strengthening the other glands such as with nose to tail eating (consuming all the organs including the brain), using a multi-glandular formula that contains the important organs and glands such as is available at traditionalfoods.org, or with organic colostrum.

The Thyroid Gland

The thyroid is regulated by the anterior portion of the pituitary gland. Often the relationship of the thyroid to the pituitary is not considered, leaving thyroid treatments ineffective. A malfunctioning thyroid also plays a role in producing tooth decay and gum disease because the thyroid along with the tiny parathyroid glands play an important role in maintaining blood calcium levels. To repair thyroid function, the anterior portion of the pituitary gland usually needs attention. A low sugar diet, glandular concentrates, organic colostrum, and herbal medicines are ways to support the anterior pituitary and thyroid. People on medications that affect their thyroid can have significant calcium problems that result in tooth decay, gum disease, or both.

Sex Glands

Excess testosterone can be linked to inflamed gums and excess levels of phosphorus in the blood stream.[23] Excess estrogen can also cause inflamed gums. These imbalances can have a multitude of causes such as not going to sleep when it's dark, eating the wrong types of foods, plastic toxins like BPA and BPH, pesticides, soy in foods, birth control pills, I.U.D., and many more.

Pancreas

When the pancreas is not working properly and fails to produce adequate amounts of enzymes we experience indigestion, belching, excessive gas, and over time, gum disease.[24] Pancreatic failure (diabetes) is intimately connected with gum disease. The pancreas can be supported by high quality pancreatic enzymes (which contain animal pancreas or extracts), herbs, enzymatically-rich foods such as fermented milk (yogurt, kefir, etc.), or fermented vegetables, green juice, and green smoothies.

Support Glandular Function Naturally

The healthy functioning of the pituitary, thyroid, sex glands, and all other glands is essential for a healthy body. This means that part of healing gum disease is helping restore balance and vitality to these glands. Prescription drugs, birth control pills, heavy metals, toxic and denatured foods, pesticides, plastics, and electromagnetic fields along with emotional stress factors can significantly influence one or several of our glands and leave us susceptible to gum disease. Conversely, supporting the health of our glands can support a faster recovery from gum disease. The secret to glandular balance is found in the sacred foods of indigenous cultures. It is the hormones and a variety of other potent substances in the animal tissues that comprise the sacred food categories of indigenous peoples around the world. Foods high in those special substances will support gland and hormone function to help heal gum recession.

A healthy diet low in sweets, consuming a variety of organs and glands from either fresh animal sources or from glandular concentrates, organic colostrum, herbal medicines, and a pituitary or hypothalamus concentrate are all ways to support the health and balance of these glands. Fermented grass-fed dairy products, animal fats, and cultured butter or ghee will also support the functions of the neuroendocrine system. Organic cow colostrum (the first milk from the animal after birth) contains precursors for all the hormones that support all the glandular functions along with growth factors to help regenerate the body, as well as immunity-building factors. Since it can be difficult to obtain a wide variety of fresh organ meats, consuming a dried organ and glandular blend from grass-fed sources mimics the practice of consuming these parts of the animal by traditional peoples around the world. Eating zinc-rich oysters and mineral-rich seaweed and shellfish can also help balance the hormonal system. Special foods and herbs can also be used if you discover your specific hormonal imbalance. Many of these nutrient-dense foods in dried form can be found at traditionalfoods.org. To obtain fresh versions, I recommend your trusted local farmer, farmers' markets, and even a well-stocked health food store.

How Sugar Imbalances Glandular Function and Contributes Significantly to Gum Disease

The extensive research of Dr. Hawkins and Dr. Page shows us that healthy teeth and gums require a balanced level of calcium and phosphorous in our blood. In order for these levels to stay in balance, we need to have at least adequate glandular function and a normally functioning autonomic nervous system. **Anything that consistently throws the glandular or nervous system out of balance can cause gum recession, as well as other conditions.**

After the last chapter which correlated high sugar intake with physical decay and deterioration, it is probably not surprising when I tell you that high intensity sweeteners (that is, anything that is very sweet), which for the sake of clarity in this chapter I will call sugar, has a powerfully detrimental effect on the functioning of the glandular system.

Dr. Page called gum disease "arthritis of the periodontium" back in 1949. More recently, researchers have found that rheumatoid arthritis patients are eight times more likely to suffer from periodontal disease than those without arthritis.[25] In case studies of several hundred people suffering from various forms of arthritis, Dr. Page found nearly all of them consumed large quantities of sugar. This is a problem because sugar seriously disturbs calcium and phosphorous metabolism. Sugar first raises the body's blood calcium and lowers blood phosphorus. When the effect of sugar wears off, a rebound effect lowers blood calcium and raises blood phosphorous.[26] A friendly reminder: low blood calcium is the precursor to gum disease.

It is easiest to think of high intensity sweeteners not as foods, but more like drugs. During his life, Dr. Melvin Page extensively investigated the effect of blood sugar fluctuations on tooth decay and gum disease. Testing blood chemistry in his laboratory, he linked fluctuating blood sugar levels with fluctuating calcium and phosphorus ratios. White sugar produces the most significant blood sugar fluctuations, which lasts five hours. Fruit sugar produces fewer fluctuations, but the blood sugar also remains out of balance for five hours. Honey causes even fewer fluctuations and blood sugar stabilizes after three hours.[27] (This is not a blanket endorsement of honey, as most honey available commercially today is from bees fed a synthetic sugar, rather than from naturally occurring pollen and nectar.) If blood sugar fluctuations become habitual, then calcium is pulled into the blood from your teeth, jaw bones, and other bones in order to stabilize it. This manifests as a systemic disease when our blood sugar remains out of control day in and day out because of poor diet and/or because of weaknesses and imbalances within the glandular system. To cure gum disease or tooth decay, our lesson from Dr. Page is to do everything possible to stabilize blood sugar levels and attain the correct ratio of calcium and phosphorous in the blood.[28]

The longer and more often our blood sugar is out of balance, the longer and more significantly the calcium and phosphorus ratios are altered. The longer and more significantly the calcium and phosphorous ratios are altered, the more damage we do to our glands, as well as to our teeth and periodontium. Regardless of whether the sugar is white sugar or sugar from fruit consumption, it still has adverse effects on our blood sugar levels.

High fructose sweeteners such as corn syrup do not offer a respite. Despite the fact that they do not affect blood sugar levels, they do affect blood fructose levels. High fructose corn syrup and synthetic sugars will disrupt calcium metabolism and definitely cause diabetes in lab animals.[29,30] If sweet foods, natural or processed, are consumed several times per day, then the alteration in blood sugar will be prolonged and consistent. Over time, this will lead to a consistent alteration of blood calcium and phosphorous levels and likely cause cavities or gum recession. **All sweet foods, no matter how natural, cause blood sugar fluctuations.** How much one's blood sugar fluctuates is related to the intensity of the sweetness. Therefore dates, or dried fruit, may cause significantly more blood sugar fluctuations than a sour green apple. If sugar or sweet foods are a part of your regular diet, particularly in large amounts, then your blood sugar level never has much time to recover to normal.

In the year 2000, the USDA estimated that the average person consumes 152 pounds of sugar per year. Of these 152 pounds, approximately 66 pounds are comprised of white sugar with the remaining 85 pounds coming from corn-derived sweeteners such as glucose, dextrose, and high fructose corn syrup.[31] In 1822, when refined sugar was a costly commodity and primarily in reach only for the wealthy, the average daily sugar consumption measured only about two teaspoons per day.[32] Today the average American consumes nearly twenty-three times more sugar, consuming forty-seven teaspoons of sugar per day, or nearly one full cup of sugar, accounting for about 580 calories per day. The diet that completely wrecked the Eskimos' teeth and gums consisted of about 1,200 calories per day from sugar. Our bodies' sugar balancing systems are not built to handle the flood of refined sugar now normally consumed. As a result, many degenerative changes take place for this reason alone or in conjunction with others. Diabetes is the chief affliction, **but the resulting mineral imbalance of the blood from excess sugar is responsible for gum disease,** dental decay, arthritis and other degenerative changes.[33]

Given that excess sugar and sweetener consumption causes an imbalance of our calcium and phosphorous levels in the blood, it is not surprising that many researchers have found correlations between periodontal disease and diabetes. In 1910, the Journal of the American Medical Association (JAMA), reported "gingivitis is an early and prominent symptom in many cases of diabetes mellitus."[34] Nearly one hundred years later, a 2008 research article in the Journal of the American Dental Association concluded that "data support the fact that periodontitis is a complication of diabetes."[35] This research confirms the findings of Dr. Page.

In a 2011 study of 1500 diabetic patients, a direct correlation between blood sugar levels and gum disease was observed.[36] The resting blood sugar increases because the body's ability to maintain a healthy blood sugar level is damaged by excess sugar consumption. This chart also shows that the worse the body's ability to handle sugar, the more severe the periodontal disease.

Type 1 gum disease is caused by chronically low blood calcium and high phosphorous levels. Excess sugar consumption, which a majority of the public is guilty of, causes low blood calcium and high blood phosphorous in the long run. Thus a primary factor of gum disease is sugar consumption, and a primary method of healing gum disease will be to follow the advice of Dr. Page and normalize our blood sugar levels.

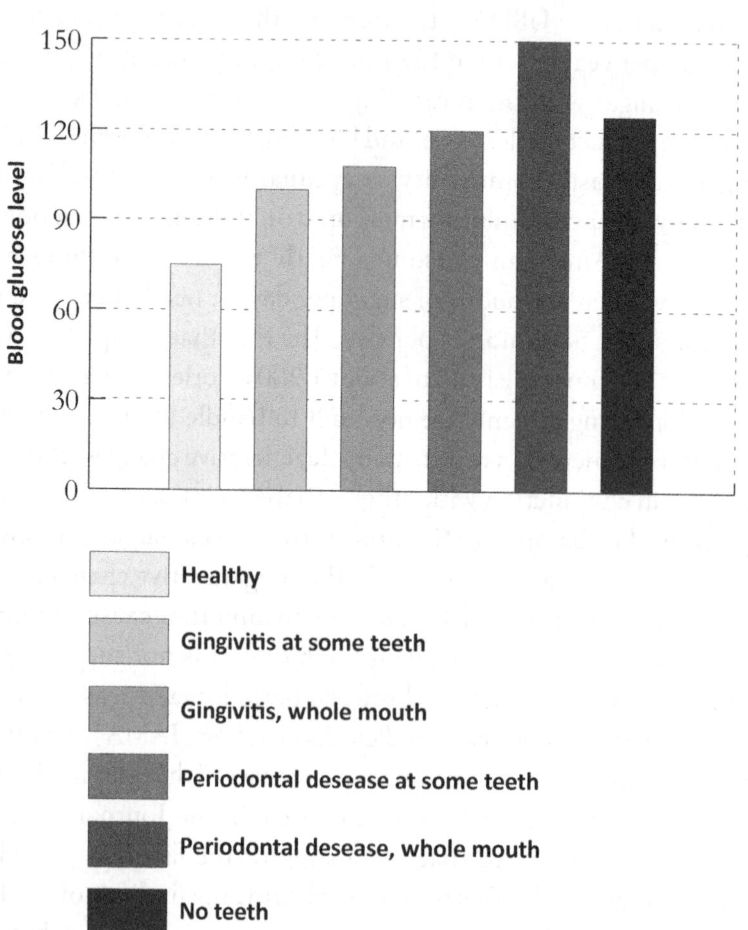

Why People Crave Sugar

With all this damning evidence about how bad sugar is for us, you might wonder why you or other people continue to consume it? Because we physically crave it. It is addicting. In a state of health, the calcium and phosphorus levels in our blood maintain a ratio of ten to four. Our bodies feel good and alive when they are healthy and balanced. When an individual's nervous system is sympathetic dominant, their blood is deficient in calcium, which serves to calm us. Because sugar increases the blood calcium temporarily, it helps the sympathetic dominant person feel good and balanced. Unfortunately after the sugar high the blood calcium soon drops, leaving the person once again in a calcium deficient state and craving even more sugar. With each bath of sugar, the body loses more and more calcium.

Host Response Explained

In the first chapter, I shared how the "host response" is what modern dentistry believes protects patients from gum disease even in the presence of bacteria. Dr. Page stated that microorganisms only become infectious after the calcium-phosphorus ratio becomes imbalanced. He wrote:

> *There exists a disturbance of the calcium-phosphorous balance when infestation of the body by microorganisms changes to infection of the body, by those same microorganisms which have been present during long periods of health.*[37]

Modern periodontology has been treating periodontal disease as if the disease was some type of surgical wound caused by microorganisms. Dentistry keeps trying to clean the wound from bacteria to promote healing. But the bacteria have always been in our mouths—**clearly gum disease is not just a wound.**

Both gum disease and tooth decay have the same root cause: a disturbance in our nervous and glandular systems as a result of eating too much sweet food and not enough fat-soluble vitamins and minerals (chiefly calcium and phosphorous).

The Real Cause of Aggressive Periodontal Disease and Pregnancy Gingivitis

Synthesizing the work from Drs. Price, Page, and Hawkins shows us the potential true cause of pregnancy gingivitis and aggressive periodontal disease. In chapter one I mentioned aggressive periodontal disease which is fast-acting gum recession that happens primarily to young people during times of rapid growth. This condition is not caused by bacteria; rather, when teenagers grow quickly during puberty, their bodies' demand for calcium, phosphorous, and other minerals increases! These teenagers succumb to Type 2 gum recession, in which alveolar bone is lost because of insufficient minerals in the diet before and during the time of rapid growth.

In similar fashion, it is common for pregnant women to develop gingivitis. While the blame is placed on hormonal changes, it is more likely that the normal hormonal changes of pregnancy increase the demand and draw of calcium from the bones so that minerals can be delivered to the growing fetus.[38] If pregnant women increase their calcium intake from natural foods, pregnancy gingivitis will drop, and both mothers and babies will be more adequately nourished.

A Common Sense Theory on the True Nature of Periodontal Disease

Our bones, including the alveolar bone, go through a process known as "bone remodeling." What happens in our mouths daily is that new bone is constantly being formed by osteoblasts (cells that help build bones), and old bone is constantly being resorbed by osteoclasts (cells that absorb bone tissue).[39] The massive chewing, biting, and clenching forces of our mouths mean that there is significant bone remodeling occurring in the alveolar bone. Daily our alveolar bone is being destroyed, and daily, the body must work hard to rebuild it. When there are not enough minerals to remodel the alveolar bone, the bone is destroyed faster than it is remodeled and rebuilt. The result is gum disease and to heal it, we will need not only to provide the quantities but also the proper proportions of the minerals our bodies need.

Chewing, Biting, and Gum Disease

Our mouths create an enormous amount of force when we chew, or clench our teeth. This force is anywhere from seventy to five hundred pounds per square inch. Our teeth are suspended in their sockets by the periodontal ligament. The periodontal ligament as well as the supporting bone acts like a shock absorber for the various chewing, biting, and clenching forces that our teeth undergo. The support beam of this shock-absorbing mesh is the alveolar bone. It is rather like

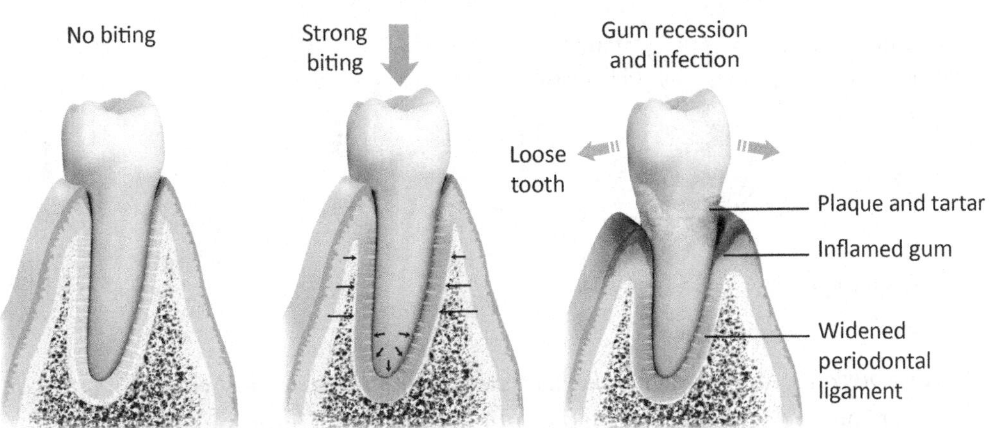

One of the symptoms of Dental Compression Syndrome, the wearing away of teeth from compressive forces of the mouth, is gum recession.[40] *As the bone is resorbed due to biting forces and a demineralized diet, the part of the alveolar bone that is the thinnest succumbs first.*

when you jump on a trampoline; there is a massive force pulling inward on the trampoline's support beams. The higher portions of the alveolar bone shown in the picture are typically lost first, perhaps because it has the most inward pulling forces and the least compressive forces (compressive force stimulates the bone rebuilding phase).

Occlusal stress plays an important role in contributing to alveolar bone loss. This can be caused by bad orthodontics, poor dental work, or other injury to the body, head, or sacrum like a car accident. Occlusion and gum recession are further discussed in Chapter 9. Author's note: orthodontic treatments such as braces and headgear that compress the maxilla (upper palate) frequently damage the body, face, and periodontium, which results in abnormal bite forces on specific teeth, or TMJ stress, both of which can contribute to gum recession. You can learn more about the dangers of orthodontics and possible alternatives at: **curegumdisease.com/orthodontics**

When there are low blood mineral levels, primarily from a poor diet, **our body enhances the bone destructive phase to raise blood calcium levels.** During this period of enhanced bone destruction, calcium is released from the bones and migrates to more vital organs. The rapid active phase of gum disease observed in the periodontal literature is likely this bone destructive phase, which is then fol-

Gum Disease is the Loss of the Alveolar Bone due to Body Activated Demineralization

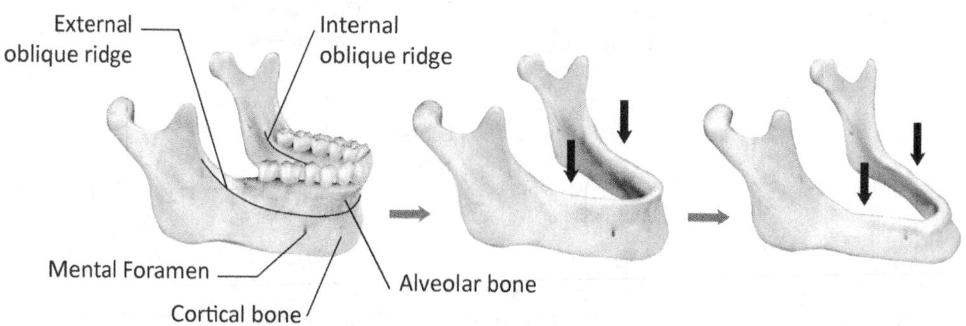

We lose our alveolar bone when the body cannot build up bone fast enough relative to how fast bone is destroyed through the natural processes of biting and chewing.

lowed by a period of remission as the body has temporarily an adequate supply of calcium. This entire time the body is in control of the resorption process.

When blood calcium levels are low the parathyroid secretes parathyroid hormone, which increases bone resorption to ensure that there is enough calcium in the blood.[41]

When the process of bone destruction exceeds the speed at which our body rebuilds bone, then the alveolar bone starts getting softer and weaker. Then, normal biting forces become like injuries to the bone. The body tries to heal the injury and it cannot. What happens when we have an injury in our body that doesn't heal, like a cut? It typically becomes infected. If the body cannot clean up or heal the damage to the alveolar bone fast enough, the area becomes infected. There is then a discharge of pus around the gums, once called pyorrhea, or in today's term, periodontitis (gum disease). This pyorrheic infection is a backup way of the body protecting itself.

Why You? Another Perspective to Consider

You may have asked this question to yourself already: why do you suffer from gum disease, while perhaps your friends or family who lead a similar lifestyle do not?

The pattern of being too active, of forcing oneself to do too much, to be an overachiever, and to go beyond one's means are characteristics of sympathetic nervous system dominance. These are not necessarily negative traits, but when overdone, can lead to imbalance. The roots of these imbalances are deep-seated emotional patterns that you may feel that you need to "run away" from. Slowing down for sympathetic-dominant types means that they may have to face uncomfortable feelings that lie beneath the surface of their incessant activity. These feelings could be a loss of love, not feeling cherished, loneliness, hatred, hostility, anger, resentment, and so on. As soon as sympathetic-dominant types slow down and start to feel an uncomfortable feeling, they immediately look for something to do, something to stimulate themselves with and rush on to the next thing rather than stay with the unpleasant feeling.

A psychological study on patients with gum disease showed that the condition is related to the "oral" character structure. This psychological pattern is something all of us have. Its roots are found in the real or perceived experience of abandonment and/or neglect in childhood and infancy.[42] The part of the infant self that was abandoned did not receive enough sweet and nourishing breast milk. As a result, the unfulfilled child attempts to regain this gratification in the adult world by consuming sweet foods. This consumption never fills the emptiness within. Eventually the body deteriorates from problems like gum disease if the addiction is not given up. Another common issue for this type of character pattern is to have longstanding agitations or aggravations in life, such as relationship conflicts and minor repetitive conflicts with authority figures like bosses or government agencies. Never feeling satiated and not having one's needs met leads to feeling angry at life, because one works hard but does not receive many rewards and rest for the hard work. Suppressed anger and rage is the key reason why we become unempowered to reach out in the world and grasp what we need.

As a part of this pattern of seeking sugar or sweet foods as a way to substitute an unfulfilled need, the individual has given up on his or her dreams. Because he or she feels like they cannot seek and find what they long for in life, a pseudo-solution like sugar or alcohol fills in the emptiness. First the emptiness was caused by the abandonment and a lack of bonding with a beloved parent in childhood. The abandonment might not be the parent literally leaving. It could be that the parent was emotionally unavailable or selectively unavailable. The abandonment becomes embedded into one's worldview. And later this emotional emptiness becomes a self-fulfilling prophecy created by the adult as the childhood pattern is subconsciously repeated over and over again by the individual's abandonment and neglect of their own hopes, dreams, and desires.

The people with whom I have collaborated who have found improvement or healing of their gum disease have been willing to stop giving up on their dreams, and start really allowing themselves to live the life that is satisfying for them. In other words, they chose to finally give themselves the nourishment that they both need and deserve.

On that note, it's time to explore much more deeply how to nourish ourselves with good food.

Know the True Nature of the Cause of Gum Disease Chapter Summary

- ❑ Healthy tissues in the mouth are a result of cells throughout the body being adequately nourished with all of the necessary vitamins, minerals, and hormones.
- ❑ A functional glandular system is critical for us to metabolize these nutrients in our food.
- ❑ Gum disease, whether it be Type 1, 2 or 3, is a result of whole body imbalances and it is not just an isolated oral problem.
- ❑ The extensive research of Dr. Hawkins and Dr. Page shows us that healthy teeth and gums require a balanced level of calcium and phosphorous in our blood. In order for these levels to stay in balance, we need to have at least adequate glandular function and a normally functioning autonomic nervous system. Anything that consistently throws the glandular or nervous system out of balance can cause gum recession, as well as other diseases.
- ❑ Sugar consumption affects our blood sugar levels. Consistent sugar consumption disrupts our body's calcium and phosphorus ratios. Over time, this results in tooth decay, gum disease, and other illnesses.
- ❑ Dr. Hawkins' saliva and calcium chart shows us that tooth decay and gum disease happens as a result of biochemical imbalances, and not bacteria.
- ❑ To regain oral health, people need to move back into the ideal range, which means finding pH balance and restoring depleted calcium and phosphorous.

4 Deficiency in Vitamins Causes Gum Disease and Restoring Those Vitamins Cures Gum Disease Naturally

Why so many of us have gum disease could not be clearer. Dr. Price's field studies demonstrate clearly that the diet most of us consume is too high in sugar and severely deficient in the vitamins and minerals our bodies need to obtain good health.

Healing gum disease is almost as simple as A, B, C, D. . . and K. But being conceptually simple does not necessarily mean it is easy to apply with our modern and denatured food supply. Conventional doctors and dietitians tell us that serious vitamin deficiencies are rare because western medicine tends to recognize vitamin deficiencies only in their most overt, extreme forms. Blinded by this overly narrow indoctrinated teaching, both dentists and periodontists today rarely consider vitamin deficiencies as the main culprit behind tooth decay or gum disease. This blindness has arisen from the post World War II mid 1900s' antibiotic revolution, in which there became a single-minded obsession with bacteria as the cause of disease. Prior to that time, rather than being taboo, it was far more common for dentists to focus on vitamins, minerals, and nutrition.

Vitamin A Deficiency and Periodontal Disease

Dr. Hawkins found that 70 percent of his patients with dental problems tested having borderline or low vitamin A levels.[1] Vitamin A plays an important role in vision, bone growth, reproduction, cell division, proper prenatal development, and cell differentiation. Vitamin A is crucial for healthy bones and, together with vitamin D, stimulates and regulates bone growth.[2] We want to stimulate bone growth because gum recession is really bone loss in the jaw.

Any impairment in liver function impedes vitamin A assimilation, so it is important that we have healthy livers. Dr. Hawkins attributed vitamin A deficiencies to the use of pasteurized butter and milk because the industrial production of butter and milk rendered them low in vitamin A.[3]

Vitamin A deficiency results in a change in epithelial tissue such as skin, mucous membranes, and gland coverings. A sensitive mucous membrane means gum tissue will be more prone to bleeding, attachment loss from scaling and root planing, and excessive redness associated with gingivitis. In addition, gum disease caused by a vitamin A deficiency results in loose teeth but tight gums.[4]

I have created a chart below of foods high in vitamin A so that you can consciously choose vitamin A-rich foods to include in your diet regularly. The foods selected are only from preformed vitamin A as retinol. Note that the Weston A. Price Foundation does recommend more than the United States Department of Agriculture's published Recommended Daily Intake, or RDI.

Obtaining Fat-Soluble Vitamin A

Recommended Intake

4,000-10,000+ IU as per the Weston A. Price Foundation

2,300-3000 IU RDI of Retinol as per the USDA

Food	Vitamin A Amount in IU
Fermented cod liver oil – 1 teaspoon	Very High
Turkey liver – 2 ounces	43,000
Beef and duck liver – 2 ounces	20,000 - 23,000
Chicken liver – 2 ounces	7,600
Fish eyes / animal eyes	Very high
Goat cheese – 3.5 ounces	1,464 -1,745
Duck egg – 1 egg	472
King salmon – 3.5 ounces	453
Butter or ghee – 1 tablespoon	350 - 391
High vitamin butter oil – 1 teaspoon	200 - 450
Egg yolk – 1 ½ yolks	333
Whole milk – 1 cup	249

In examining this list, you will see that liver is the most concentrated source of fat-soluble vitamin A. The magic of liver in relation to healing gum disease in part is its high vitamin A content, and in part its mineral and B vitamin content.

B Vitamins and Gum Disease

Vitamin B1 – Thiamine

Beriberi was the first nutritional deficiency disease recognized by the modern western medical world. Beriberi is caused by a thiamine deficiency that occurs in a diet that is composed almost exclusively of white rice. Oral symptoms of a B1 deficiency include hypersensitivity and erosion of the soft tissues in the mouth.[5] Other symptoms include malaise, loss of appetite, gastrointestinal disturbance, heart palpitations, and shortness of breath. Alcohol abuse can also impair the body's ability to absorb vitamin B1 and thereby cause beriberi, also contributing to gum problems.

Foods High in B1

Basic Intake 1.1-1.2 mg (RDI)

Food	B1 or Niacin in Milligrams
Pork – various cuts – 3.5 ounces	0.8 –1.0 mg
Macadamia nuts, pine nuts, sunflower seeds – ½ cup	0.3 – 0.45 mg
Trout, salmon, tuna – 3.5 ounces	0.1 – 0.43 mg
Navy, black, mung beans, or lentils – 3.5 ounces	0.17 – 0.44 mg
Green peas – 3.5 ounces	0.28 mg

Most of the nutrient values in the vitamin charts are for cooked foods. An interesting fact is that cooked brown rice and cooked white rice have nearly the same amount of vitamin B1. We often hear that brown rice is superior to white in nutritional value; however, it may not be that simple because white rice actually has more B vitamins, while brown has more minerals.[6,7]

Vitamin B2 – Riboflavin

Dr. Hawkins believed that excess consumption of refined carbohydrates (such as white flour and sugar) cause a deficiency in salivary amylase. When this digestive enzyme is deficient, starches are not properly broken down by the saliva. Food-based vitamins B1 and B2 can help correct this condition. A 1936 study found a B2-deficient diet created mouth lesions and gingivitis in rhesus monkeys.[8] Therefore one can infer that vitamin B2 plays an important role in gum health and in the prevention of gingivitis. The following is not a complete list, but rather, a highlight of foods that are very high in B2. Note that liver once again supplies superior quantities. Animal hearts and game meat also contain modest amounts of B2.

Foods High in B2

Basic Intake: 1.1-1.3mg per day (RDI) [9]

Food	B2 or Riboflavin in Milligrams
Lamb, beef, pork, chicken, turkey liver – 2 ounces	1-3 mg
Lamb, beef, pork kidney – 2 ounces	1 mg
Mackerel – 3 ounces	0.5 mg
Almonds – 1 ounce	0.23 mg

Vitamin B3 – Niacin

Pellagra was once endemic in the southern United States and is caused by a vitamin B3 deficiency. It was primarily caused by eating corn that had not been nixtamalized. Nixtamalization is the cooking and soaking of corn with highly alkaline calcium-rich lime to release vitamins and minerals. The best-known symptoms of pellagra are the "three Ds" of dermatitis, dementia, diarrhea, and if left untreated, pellagra causes death. Pellagra also results in inflammation, redness, soreness, and irritation of the mouth.[10] One of the first signs of niacin deficiency is painful gingivitis and inflammation of the gingival lining.[11]

The effect of a lack of B vitamins over long periods of time might be responsible for cases of loose teeth due to gum disease.[12] Mild or sub-acute cases of pellagra have been frequently mistaken for gum disease. In these instances, dental cleaning or surgery alone will fail to improve the condition because descaling or surgical treatment does not address the root cause of gum disease.

Foods High in B3

Basic Intake: 14-16mg per day (RDI)

Food	B3 or Niacin in Milligrams
Chicken, tuna, sturgeon – 3.5 ounces	11-12 mg
Beef liver – 2 ounces	10 mg
Mackerel, salmon, swordfish – 3.5 ounces	9-10 mg
Pork meat – 3.5 ounces	8-10 mg
Red meat: top sirlion / ribeye – 3.5 ounces	8 mg
Chicken / turkey liver – 2 ounces	8 mg
Marmite – yeast extract – 1 teaspoon	5.8 mg
Anchovies – 1 ounce	5.6 mg
Various mushrooms – 3.5 ounces	3-4 mg
Brewer's yeast – 1 teaspoon	2.5 mg

Vitamin B5 – Pantothenic Acid, B6, B7, and Choline

None of the sources I considered pointed to either B5 or B6 deficiencies as significant causes of periodontal disease. Nevertheless, since the other members of the B vitamin complex are so crucial to gum health, it is likely that vitamins B5 and B6 also play some role that has not yet been clearly identified. These lists can be used to fine-tune your diet.

Foods High in B5 – Mushrooms, particularly shiitake and white button, are high in B5. Other good sources include oily fish, bird eggs, red meat, pork, chicken, turkey, liver, nixtamalized corn, and sunflower seeds.[13]

Foods High in B6 – Fish, in particular tuna and salmon, turkey, chicken, pork, red meat, animal livers, nixtamalized corn, and sunflower seeds are all high in B6.[14]

High in B7 (Biotin) – Eggs and liver.[15]

High in Choline – Egg yolk, liver, kidneys, brain, and fish eggs. Seafood, broccoli, and Brussels sprouts have less, yet still modest amounts of choline.[16]

Vitamin B9 – Folate

Folate is the B vitamin that occurs naturally in food, while folic acid is the synthetic version of the vitamin. Some studies have connected low dietary folate levels with periodontal disease.[17] Dietary folate can help with reducing inflammation associated with gum disease.

Food Folate – Vitamin B9

Basic Intake: 400 micrograms (mcg) (RDI)

Food	B9 or Folate in Micrograms
Chicken, turkey, duck liver – 2 ounces	300-386 mcg
Chicken / turkey giblets – 1.5 ounces	168 mcg
Black or mung beans, chickpeas, lentils – 3.5 ounces	150-170 mcg
Asparagus, okra, spinach – 3.5 ounces	135-150 mcg
Beef, pork, lamb liver – 2 ounces	140 mcg
Broccoli, brussels sprouts – 3.5 ounces	100 mcg
Romaine lettuce – 1 cup, shredded	64 mcg

Vitamin B12

Since gum disease is a result of various vitamin deficiencies including those in the B vitamin complex, it's not surprising that scientific studies would find a connection between anemia, periodontal disease, and B12 deficiencies.[18 19]

Vitamin B12

Basic Intake: 2.4 micrograms (mcg)(RDI)

Food	B12 in Micrograms
Clams – 1.75 ounces	50 mcg
Lamb, turkey, beef, pork, chicken liver – 1.75 ounces	15-45 mcg
Octopus – 1.75 ounces	18 mcg
Oysters – 1.75 ounces	15 mcg
Mussels – 1.75 ounces	10 mcg
Mackerel, herring – 1.75 ounces	9 mcg
Crab – 3.5 ounces	9.8 mcg
Beef / various cuts – 3.5 ounces	6 mcg
Bluefish, salmon, bass – 3.5 ounces	4 mcg
Fish eggs / caviar – 1 tablespoon	3.2 mcg

Not all B vitamins have a proven direct association with gum health, but we know that B vitamins work best together. In general, consuming high quality animal foods from the land and the sea, both the flesh meat and the organs, is a good strategy to obtain adequate levels of B vitamins. This information is incorporated into the more specific daily dietary guidelines found in chapter eight, which is all about healing gum disease with food.

Obtaining B Vitamins from Food

Two ounces per day of beef liver provides the following percentage of RDI for the nutrients listed below:

Food	Vitamin A	B1	B2	B3	B5	B6	B9	B12
Beef liver	356%	8%	105%	50%	50%	30%	36%	658%

Proteins from healthy animal foods provide reasonable amounts of B vitamins. Liver is the B vitamin super food, and consuming liver regularly will carry you well on your way towards an adequate daily B vitamin intake. You may select liver from not only beef, but from any healthy, farm-raised animal such as pork, lamb, chicken, and turkey.

Grass-fed Liver Intake
2+ ounces of fresh liver 2-4+ times per week or
1-3 teaspoons of dried powdered liver 2-4 times per week

For those who do not enjoy eating liver or find it difficult to find high quality liver, the best alternative may be a liver powder supplement. Liver is revered as a sacred healing food in cultures around the world and belongs in any gum healing program. Once you begin consuming liver regularly and start feeling the positive effects, you'll understand why liver is one of the most valued and sacred food items that there is. Freeze dried liver is available at traditionalfoods.org.

Low Income Considerations

In parts of this book, I recommend buying supplements and certain foods that I envision are affordable for most people, but I acknowledge that this is not so for everyone. I understand that some items may be financially out of reach for some people. To remedy this, I will provide a food list and dietary guide for healing gum disease on an extremely low budget at curegumdisease.com/budget.

Vitamin C Deficiency and Gum Disease

Mild and sub-acute vitamin C deficiencies contribute to periodontal disease.[20,21] The importance of vitamin C to the gingival and alveolar bone has been amply demonstrated in human and animal experiments.[22]

Scurvy was once a common cause of suffering and death among sailors and was a significant hindrance to long distance sea travel from the fifteenth to early twentieth centuries. The cause of this malady was a severe and prolonged vitamin C deficiency. Symptoms of less extreme scurvy include periodontal disease, general aches and pains, susceptibility to infections, and capillary fragility. More extreme scurvy results in spongy and bleeding gums, loose teeth, sore joints, shortness of breath, loss of weight, and pseudo paralysis.[23] Since many people with gum disease have scorbutic symptoms, it might be useful to know briefly what the sailors ate and what they did not eat that caused these health problems.

Historically, the diet of sailors consisted of food that would last a long time without refrigeration. They ate salted beef, pork, and fish, as well as approximately one pound per day of hardtack, which were biscuits made of whole wheat flour, water, and salt, baked several times to remove all moisture. At the time of the Spanish Armada (1588), sailors were allowed one gallon of beer per day, which stored better than fresh water that would soon grow algae in barrels. This diet was completely devoid of any source of vitamin C from a fresh or raw plant source.

Vitamin C deficiency causes the degeneration of the intercellular substances of teeth and bones. Bone tissues then lose their calcium and loose teeth result. Vitamin C deficiency contributes to rapid bone resorption and the reduction of enzymes that support normal mouth flora.[24]

Signs of vitamin C deficiency include loose teeth without infection and bright red, swollen gingival tissues caused by the suppression of collagen synthesis.[25] Vitamin C and calcium work together, as vitamin C cannot maintain bone integrity without a calcium supply.[26]

Many dental scholars believed that gingivitis was a result of vitamin C deficiency and that the absence of vitamin C predisposed people to gum disease. This predisposition is avoided by daily adequate ingestion of vitamin C-containing foods.[27] Some evidence points to the reason for vitamin C's effectiveness being its ability to help maintain a balanced blood calcium and phosphorous ratio.[28, 29]

In taking vitamin C from food or supplements you may not notice an immediate health improvement because the blood must maintain a stable level of vitamin C. But over time, you will likely notice a positive difference, as vitamin C is important for so many of the body's functions.

Oranges are included in the list for information, but because they contain so much sugar per orange—about 15 percent of one's daily sugar intake in a single orange—it is not realistic or healthy for people with gum disease to consume large quantities of oranges. This is because excess sugar consumption, as discussed in the previous chapter, is a primary cause of calcium and phosphorous imbalances, and blood sugar levels are directly correlated with the severity of gum disease.

Unlike most mammals, humans do not have the ability to make ascorbic acid and must obtain vitamin C from their diet. Vitamin C is thus considered an essential dietary component. Most vitamin C supplements on the market are synthetic forms of vitamin C. Only a few companies sell true vitamin C that comes from nature such as from berries, or cherries. Many of the vitamin C products on the market contain overt or hidden synthetic ascorbic acid.

Real food vitamin C is not the same as isolated ascorbic acid. Ninety percent of ascorbic acid manufactured for the vitamin supplement industry is produced in one factory and is usually extracted from genetically modified (GM) corn. Isolated

Vitamin C in Food

Basic Intake: 75-90mg (RDI)

Food	Vitamin C in Milligrams
High vitamin C powder from organic acerola – ¼ teaspoon	250 mg
Guava – 1 fruit – 5 grams of sugar	126 mg
Papaya – 1 cup cubed – 8 grams of sugar	87 mg
Parsley – 1 cup raw	80 mg
Kiwi – 1 medium – 7 grams of sugar	70 mg
Orange – 1 large – 14 grams of sugar	60-83 mg
Organic camu camu (depends on brand) – ¼ teaspoon	60 mg
Kale – 1 cup	53 mg
Red, yellow, green pepper – 1 ounce	50 mg
Broccoli – ½ cup	50 mg
Kohlrabi, brussels sprouts, cauliflower – ½ cup	35 mg
Lemon – 1 regular	31 mg
Strawberry – 4 medium – 4 grams of sugar	28 mg
Potato – 1 whole	20 mg
Milk – 4 cups	19 mg
Persimmon – 1 fruit	16 mg
Tomato – 1 medium	15 mg
Raw sauerkraut – ¼ cup	9 mg
Adrenal gland	High / unknown

Dried rose hips, sometimes recommended for vitamin c supplementation, often do not contain too much vitamin C unless freshly picked.

ascorbic acid lacks the cofactors that naturally exist with vitamin C found in food. It is a manufactured "food supplement" of the laboratory and does not resemble any plant that grew in the soil. Therefore, synthetic vitamin C works in the body more like a drug than a food. That means it can have therapeutic drug-like uses, but for our purposes here of longer-term use, it is best to consume nutrients as produced by nature in whole foods. Synthetic vitamin C is in fact not easily metabolized and may mostly result in "expensive urine."[30]

Because of the importance of a whole-food source of vitamin C complex to overall health and well being, I tested a variety of products available to find the highest potency, most absorbable organic form of vitamin C. Many, but not all companies avoid using the highest quality vitamin C from food because of the expense. The website traditionalfoods.org offers a nutrient-dense *High Vitamin C* product which is purely low-temperature dried organic acerola cherry juice powder.

Before following any dietary advice or purchasing any recommended products in this book, please review my product disclaimer in Appendix A.

Vitamin C Therapeutic Dosage

Remember each person is very different, and having some type of energetic test to determine your optimal dose from a health provider is optimal. Alternatively, take the amount that feels good to you! And as a reminder, each individual is unique. I am offering you choices to help you find what will work for you. I suggest taking one or more days off per week of most vitamins or supplements just to give your body a chance to recalibrate. Each person is different, so use your best judgment and seek nutritional help where appropriate.

Recommended Vitamin C Intake for Acute Imbalances
800-1,400 mg of natural, food-based vitamin C per day 4-6 days per week
For example:
⅔–2 teaspoons of High Vitamin C powder per day 4-6 days per week

Maintenance Dose

This refers to when your body is in balance and you want to help maintain balance. A modest consumption of High Vitamin C powder will help make sure you have more than an adequate amount of vitamin C.

Recommended Vitamin C Intake for Maintenance
¼-½ teaspoon of High Vitamin C Powder 4-5 days per week and/or
200–300mg Vitamin C daily from food

Example ideas for consuming vitamin C from food:

- ☐ Drinking 2-4 cups of raw vegetable juice daily, which includes parsley (recipe in food section). Two bunches of raw parsley contains roughly 230 mg of vitamin C.

- ☐ 2 cups of cooked broccoli has 200mg of vitamin C. (Note: broccoli is a member of the brassica genus and frequent consumption may not be good for everyone because of its goitrogenic properties.)
- ☐ 2 cups of cooked kale – 100mg of vitamin C.
- ☐ 1 guava has 126 mg of vitamin C.
- ☐ 1 kiwi has 70mg of vitamin C (kiwis are sweet—use in moderation).

Note: I don't recommend consuming too many sweet foods to obtain vitamin C.

Vitamin D

Vitamin D is a steroid hormone originally identified for its ability to prevent skeletal deformities referred to as rickets. Edward Mellanby, the British researcher who contributed to the discovery of vitamin D, extensively researched nutrition and tooth decay with his wife, May. Their feeding experiments on dogs proved gum disease can be both produced and prevented under lab conditions. Dietary changes profoundly affected the development of the alveolar bones and soft tissues of the mouth. Diets rich in vitamins A and D led to healthy, sound, and normal oral tissues and bone, while diets deficient in fat-soluble vitamins A and D led to advanced periodontal disease reported as deep pockets containing pus, along with resorption of the alveolar bone.[31]

The sacrifice these laboratory dogs made for the cause of human health sadly has not changed the course of dental history. Instead of learning these lessons, human beings, pets, and farm animals continue to participate as unwitting test subjects in a grand uncontrolled dietary experiment of eating industrially processed and toxic fast foods. This has led to painful gum disease, tooth decay, and other degenerative problems. May Mellanby conclusively demonstrated that changes to the alveolar bones are due to a lack of vitamin D in the diet and gum tissue. She reported that other negative soft tissue changes can be attributed to a deficiency in vitamin A.[32] These experiments furthermore showed that optimum amounts of vitamins A and D during the growing years led to a strong periodontium that is less susceptible to periodontal disease later in life.

Without vitamin D, we simply cannot utilize calcium well.[33] Vitamin D does not only help us assimilate calcium, but it also helps us maintain optimum levels of other minerals including iron, magnesium, phosphorus, and zinc. A recent meta-analysis of twenty-four excellent vitamin D studies carried out over the past ninety years showed that the average rate of dental cavities was reduced by between 47-54 percent by the administration of vitamin D.[34] Due to the fact that bone loss is a major component of periodontal disease, it makes sense that

optimum vitamin D levels have a massive and substantial impact over time on gum health. There are well-established connections between low vitamin D levels and periodontal disease.[35] Calcium utilization can double within two weeks by the administration of vitamin D and can be lost in about the same amount of time by abstaining from it.[36]

We need fat-soluble vitamins A, D, and K2 for optimum production of osteocalcin, the protein responsible for deposition of calcium and phosphorous into our bones.[37] Dr. Price found that his patients suffered from tooth decay because modern diets are severely lacking in fat-soluble vitamins. To cure gum disease, we must add these vitamins back into our diets.

Vitamin D levels in Foods

1,800-2,000 IU per day as per Dr. Hawkins
600-800 IU as per the RDI

Food	Vitamin D Amount in IU
Fermented cod liver oil – 1 teaspoon	high
X-Factor Gold™ high vitamin butter oil – 1 teaspoon	high
Tilapia (wild) – 3.5 ounces	1,800
Chum salmon (Dog, Keta, or Calico) – 3.5 ounces	1,300
Herring – 3.5 ounces	1,100
Wild sockeye / King salmon – 3.5 ounces	760-996
Sockeye salmon – 3.5 ounces	763
Pastured duck egg – 1 egg[38]	720
Halibut, trout – 3.5 ounces	600
Salmon, mackerel, sardine – 3.5 ounces	335-480
Canned sardines, cod – 3.5 ounces	280
Oysters – 6	270
Pastured lard / tallow – 3.5 ounces	100-250*
Animal blood - pastured or wild – 3.5 ounces	100-250*
Shrimp – 3.5 ounces	172
Chicken egg – 1 egg (conventional / pastured)	18 / 136-200
Tilapia – farm raised – 3.5 ounces	150
Butter – 3.5 ounces	56
Milk, conventional – 4 cups	40
Beef liver conventional – 1 ounce	10-15
Lard conventional – 1 tablespoon	14

Seafood is an excellent source of vitamin D and fish liver is the highest source. For purists, eating oily fish and fish livers would be a good means to obtain plenty of vitamin D without ingesting cod liver oil. For vegetarians, consuming moderate amounts of butter and chicken eggs will not likely provide adequate quantities of fat-soluble vitamin D. However, adding Green Pasture's™ high vitamin butter oil, and free range duck eggs would more than likely ensure for plenty of vitamin D.

In feeding trials, bacon fat did not produce the same anti-cavity effect as suet did (beef fat from cow fat deposits).[39] It is unclear how effective lard from pastured pigs will be in reversing gum disease. Animal blood from healthy animals is a traditional food and has vitamin D or vitamin D-like factors that are potent for healing tooth decay, gum disease, or other deficiency diseases.

Vitamin A and D Supplements vs. Food

There are many studies warning of adverse health effects of too much fat-soluble vitamins A and D in the diet. Most of these studies are the result of studying vitamins A and D independently and from synthetic supplements, not whole foods. I recommend only food-based forms of these vitamins to be sure our bodies can metabolize them properly. There are dozens and perhaps hundreds of forms of vitamin D, but only three major types are considered most important to humans.[40] The only way to get the full spectrum of vitamin D with all the natural co-factors is from food.

Cod Liver Oil together with Butter to Remineralize Jaw Bones and Teeth

Dr. Weston A. Price administered a mixture of butter oil and cod liver oil to reduce tooth decay by about 90 percent among his patients.[41] In a recent study, these same oils mixed with kelp powder provided a significant reduction in gum bleeding and pocket depth (see page 179 for more about the study).

Not all cod liver oils are alike. Commercial cod liver oil production includes alkali refining, bleaching, winterization which removes saturated fats, and deodorization which removes toxins but also vitamins A and D.[42] Because the vitamins are connected to both the pigments and the odors, the oil refining process destroys most of the fat-soluble vitamins A and D. Most of the cod liver oils for sale in brick-and-mortar stores do not have any of their natural vitamin D intact.[43]

Even the best available store-bought cod liver oils use artificial D_3.[44] The cod liver oil labels do not tell us this, but vitamin D in cod liver oil is removed during the distillation process, and synthetic vitamin D is added back later. Most cod liver oils also have a fractionated form of vitamin E added as a preservative. Some people taking larger doses of store-bought cod liver oil have suffered allergic responses (including warts and headaches) to the d-alpha tocopherol preservative added to most commercial cod liver oils. Because of the distillation process, there is not much of a fishy taste in store-bought cod liver oil. But the key benefit of the cod liver oil to combat alveolar bone loss is the fat-soluble vitamin D, and commercial varieties just do not have it in its natural form.

Green Pasture™ produces cod liver oil made by the fermentation of livers. This is a historical process that has been practiced for hundreds of years. In the past, fishermen in Norway would remove the cods' livers during the winter fishing months and store them in barrels.[45] When the weather warmed up, the livers fermented or aged and released their precious oil. The process of aging the livers is similar to how cured meats, cold-smoked salmon, and hard cheeses are made. The aging process breaks down the cod liver proteins and releases the oil in the livers. Historically, cod liver oil made this way has drawn mixed reviews because of its strong taste. However, this strong cod liver oil was considered very medicinal. A small percentage of people either find the flavor disagreeable or find their stomachs too sensitive and cannot take it; in general most people tolerate the ½ or more teaspoon per day. This cod liver oil contains all of the cod liver's vitamin D intact because the process utilizes fermentation rather than heat distillation for extraction. To purchase fermented cod liver oil, you can go to codliveroilshop.com.

Cod Liver Oil Dosage for Fat-Soluble Vitamins A and D
¼-½ teaspoon 2-3 times per day 5-6 days per week for a total of ½-1½ teaspoons per day

Cod Liver Oil Must Be Taken together with Butter

Cod liver oil has a positive synergistic effect with high vitamin butter oil. High vitamin butter oil was produced by Dr. Price by centrifuging cream of very nutrient rich grass-fed cows milked during the time of rapid new growth. Dr. Price separated and concentrated the oil from the cream via centrifuge. This separation means that correctly made butter oil is more concentrated than ghee (clarified butter). Dr. Price believed that butter fat protected against natural irritants found in all cod liver oils. Therefore, any consumption of cod liver oil should be done in the context of a diet that contains butter (or ghee or butter oil, or cream). Preferably dairy fat should be taken at the same time with the cod liver oil. For people who cannot tolerate any dairy products, even butter, butter oil, or ghee (which does not contain casein or lactose), then my suggestion is to consume cod liver oil with fish eggs or bone marrow.

Optimizing Cod Liver Oil Dosage

The optimum dose of cod liver oil for you will depend on many factors, including your status of the fat-soluble vitamins A and D, the foods in your diet, your weight, the climate where you live, your level of sun exposure, and overall health. While cod liver oil is in fact a whole food, some still refer to it as a supplement, because it comes in a bottle. Not every supplement mentioned in this book is right for everybody. The best way to know if a supplement is right for you is to work with a trusted health care practitioner who can use an energetic testing paradigm to determine the right supplements and right dose for you. If you do not have someone to work with, start with a small dose and work up. **Please review the product disclaimer at end of the book before taking or buying any products.**

Cod Liver Oil Alternatives

Green Pasture™ also sells an excellent skate liver oil and butter oil. Both of these "supplements" contain vitamin D as well. If cod liver oil is not right for you, you can replace your cod liver oil dose with skate liver oil or butter oil. These oils can be found at codliveroilshop.com.

> **Cod Liver Capsule dosage:** 2½ of *Green Pasture's™ cod liver oil capsules* equals about a quarter teaspoon.

Avoid Synthetic Vitamin D2

Synthetic fat-soluble vitamins should only be used briefly or under the care of a health practitioner. Synthetic vitamins act like drugs in the body and seem to have many unintended effects. Be especially careful with synthetic D2 supplements or foods containing synthetic D2.[46] I do not recommend this path to avoiding cod liver oil or skate liver oil without a good reason to do so.

Weston Priced Activator X and Vitamin K2

In his historic travels Dr. Price visited the Swiss Alps in June and witnessed that the natives of the Loetschental "thank[ed] the kind Father for evidence of his Being in the life-giving qualities of butter and cheese when the cows eat the grass near the snow line."[47] The evidence of his Being, Weston Price determined, is a hormone similar to vitamin D which he called activator X. Dr. Price theorized, "There must be some food substance that is not adequately provided in modern nutrition . . ."[48] He thought this because skeletons of indigenous people show perfect bone growth and immunity to tooth decay. The most important thing about activator X rich foods, particularly really good dairy fat, is that it helps root teeth firmly in the alveolar bone.

To Summarize Dr. Price's words, here is where you find activator X:

1. Butterfat
2. Fish eggs
3. Animal organs and animal fat (grass-fed)*
4. Milk (highest when animals are on native grasses) [49]

Dr. Price's emphasis of activator X is that it is a substance that helps with growth and reproduction and that it comes from animal fats. Milk and fish eggs are reproductive foods and both fish eggs and butter are both high in fat.

** Not all animal fats and organs are high in activator X. For it to be present, the animal must be consuming grasses and plants that are rapidly growing, and some tissues will have more of the growth and regenerative enhancing activator X than others.*

Clarifying Vitamin K2 and Activator X-Rich Foods That Stop Gum Disease

There has been some very interesting research, which states that activator X is vitamin K2.[50] While the evidence is compelling, the conclusions of high K2 foods to eat, in general, do not match very well with the sacred foods of cultures across the globe. In addition, there has become an over focus on vitamin K2 dietary supplements, which has wrongly led people to choose supplements over real foods like grass-fed butter. In order to obtain the vitamin K2-rich foods that will help reverse gum disease, a deeper consideration of vitamin K2 is required.

K vitamins are a part of a class of compounds called quinones. Natural quinones form a class of pigments that range in color from yellow to black.[51] These biological pigments are found in bacteria, fungi, and in some arthropods, including grasshoppers, ants, bees, wasps, cicadas, spiders, scorpions, crayfish, lobsters, and prawns; and in echinoderms such as sea urchins, starfish, and sea cucumber.[52]

Many well-known vitamins are forms of quinones. For example vitamin K2 is menaquinone, vitamin K1 is phylloquinone, and vitamin K3 is naphthoquinone.

Coenzyme Q10 is also called ubiquinone; the Q stands for quinone. A new vitamin-like compound is being talked about called PQQ, which is related to the B vitamin complex and stands for pyrroloquinoline quinone.

There is no doubt that Dr. Price's activator X is a quinone, a class of quinones, or is related to quinones. Activator X also acts in the body like a hormone. So the special vitamin-rich foods we are looking for are going to be rich in animal hormones and quinone pigments. That means they are going to be found in the animal fats and have pigments.

Vitamin K2 food lists are difficult to interpret for special vitamin-rich foods that stop gum disease and tooth decay, because vitamin K2 has at least ten different forms consisting of both plant and animal nature. For example, there is vitamin K2-MK4, K2-MK5, K2-MK6, and all the way to K2-MK-13. Another problem is vitamin K2 test results do not directly correspond with traditional foods that should be high in activator X; for example, pepperoni, frankfurters, and rotisserie chicken are all high in vitamin K2-MK4, while traditional foods of the Eskimos such as seal oil, whale oil, and whitefish eggs test extremely low in K2-MK4.[53] And not all foods reported to be high in vitamin K2 fit the requirement of sacred foods, because they do not contain animal fats. Natto is very high in K2-MK7, which is a bacterially produced quinone found by traditionally fermenting soybeans. While I think natto is a fine probiotic-rich side dish, it is not the type of animal tissues we are looking for to obtain optimal gum health and tissue healing.

Sacred Foods High in Activator X/"K2"

Because the food lists for vitamin K2 do not reflect special food groups exactly, for the purpose of clarity, I will not refer to the vitamin simply as vitamin K2. Foods high in activator X / "K2" are the very same foods that indigenous groups considered sacred.

1. Grass-fed dairy fat, like butter and ghee
2. Organs and glands from land animals (grass-fed and harvested during the time of rapid growth)
3. Fat, organs, and glands from sea foods
4. Insects

Some "K2"-rich foods are going to have more bone regenerative abilities than others. A fascinating discovery is that cheese and cultured dairy are very high in K2-MK9.[54] This leads me to the conclusion that the best source of activator X is not just grass-fed butter, but **cultured** grass-fed butter, **cultured** ghee, or **cultured** butter oil from the time of rapid growth. Traditional ghee, which originates from India, is made with cultured dairy. Traditionally-made cheese and soured or cultured grass-fed milk are also generally high in K2-MK9. This again implies that the bacterial processing of foods may impart special unknown healing qualities to certain foods.

Non-Dairy Activator X/"K2"

A variety of organ meats from animals grazing on their native diets harvested during the period of rapid growth could be high in vitamin activator X / "K2." Animal organs that correspond with fertility in some references include thyroid gland, stomach and intestinal lining, adrenal gland, reproductive organs, bone marrow, and animal blood. Fertility enhancing sea foods that are pigment-rich are fish eggs, sea urchin, and sea cucumber. There are also likely many other activator X-rich sea foods including the colorful innards of crab and lobster. If you cannot tolerate dairy foods, then my specific suggestions for foods to help with setting your teeth firmly into the alveolar bone are fish eggs and bone marrow, as these seem to be the most easily obtained and most likely to create the desired results.

It is optimal to consume these foods fresh, if you can obtain them. But if you have a hard time finding them or eating them, then both grass-fed bone marrow and grass-fed multi-glandular dried mix are available at traditionalfoods.org.

Avoid Synthetic Vitamin K2

While synthetic MK-4 and MK-7 may have specific nutraceutical uses, I have heard and read of a few alarming cases which suggest that these products should be regularly used only with great care or under supervision of a health professional, because they can easily change the calcium / phosphorus ratio in a way that is not intended. The conclusion I have drawn is that synthetic vitamin supplementation, taken over time, can have unintended and possibly negative consequences.

Butter for Activator X/"K2"

Activator X is a bone-remineralizing, ligament strengthening force that can remineralize oral tissues. It makes sense to include ample amounts of this in our diets. To identify its activator X/"K2" presence, take note of the pigment of butter. The period of rapid growth for grass occurs anywhere from May through September, depending on the particular climate. The more yellow and orange the summer butter, the more vitamin-rich it likely is. Activator X-rich butter is a factor of the soil, the time of the year, the breed of the animal, and the types of grasses, herbs, and legumes consumed. Grass-fed butter is not always rich in activator X, but only rich during seasons when animals graze on grass undergoing rapid new growth.

Dr. Price found that activator X-rich butter could heal rickets and that it brought blood serum calcium and phosphorous ratios toward normal.[55] In practical experiments as well as with lab animals, Dr. Price found that combining cod liver oil with yellow summer butter created a positive synergistic effect. The bottom line is yellow butter is essential to healing gum disease.

Fat Soluble Activator X/"K2" Foods

High Activator X Foods
Raw butter or ghee from cows that eat rapidly growing green grass
Raw cream from dairy animals eating rapidly growing green grass
Fish eggs
X-Factor high vitamin butter oil

Likely to Contain Activator X
Bone marrow
Skate liver oil
The mustard and tomalley (innards) of crab and lobster
Sea urchin and sea cucumber
Thyroid, stomach lining, intestines, and animal blood when the animal
eats rapidly growing grass
Traditional cheeses from grass-fed animals
Goose or duck liver
Small amounts in grass-fed eggs

Activator X / "K2" Dosage

1+ teaspoon 2-3 times per day of spring/summer grass-fed butter or ghee (1-1½ tablespoons daily / cultured is better than regular) or
1-3+ teaspoons of wild caught fish eggs per day or
¼ teaspoon 2-3 times per day of high vitamin butter oil (½-¾ teaspoons daily) or
1+ tablespoon of bone marrow or 1-2 teaspoons of marrow powder

The best butter to use is raw grass-fed butter. Water buffalo, which are used in Africa and India, seem to produce a high activator X and higher vitamin D butterfat. Raw butter is better than pasteurized because it has more healing effects on the body.[56] The effectiveness of the spring / summer grass-fed butter on remineralizing body tissues varies widely depending on what types of grasses the cows eat and the quality of soil the grasses are growing in.

Cod Liver Oil and Activator X/"K2" Dosage Summary

Recently I have given you separate dosage suggestions for cod liver oil and activator X/"K2" so that you can understand how to bring those elements individually into your diet. It is vital to mix cod liver oil with activator X/"K2" for optimal results. Instead of taking cod liver oil and butter oil dietary supplements or foods separately, you can purchase them premixed as the Blue Ice™ Royal Blend, available at codliveroilshop.com

¼-½ teaspoon Blue Ice™ Royal Blend 2-3 times per day (½-1½ teaspoons per day / 6-8 capsules) or
½-1 teaspoon of real cod liver oil per day (make sure to take with 1-3 teaspoons of butter or ghee, skate liver oil can be used to replace cod liver oil)

High Nutrient Butter Sources:

Local raw butter – Sources for local butter from grass-fed animals are available at realmilk.com. Yellow butter is available from local sources during the spring and summer after the cows eat rapidly growing green grass. You can save high vitamin butter for the winter by freezing it.

Commercial pasteurized butter – Pasteurization damages the butter's quality so it is not ideal, but it does not destroy activator X/"K2." There are numerous store brands of organic and grass-fed butter. Certified organic dairy must be on pasture for at least four months of the year, and have at least 30 percent of their total food intake must be from pasture.[57] The feed that is not hay or pasture is organic grains, which can be both corn and soy, and which are not native to the cows' diet. Because of the wide range of grass and types of feeds in the diet of a cow that is producing organic dairy, there is a wide variety in quality of organically labeled butters. Some companies do the minimum, while others do far more. As you can imagine, a very high grass diet is ideal. And the traditional method for keeping cows fed in the winter time is with dried grasses from the summer time (hay). But nearly exclusive grass-feeding without year-round pasture costs more than grains and the output of the milk can be less. Some butters are grass-fed and not even labeled. And there are grass-fed butters that are very high quality but not certified organic. Another factor in the butter quality is how the butter is made, and the pasteurization process that is used. People who eat well can have a more sensitive palate, so in the end, let taste be your guide as to the quality of the butter. If it feels good, tastes great, and digests well, it's probably a good butter. But, the only way to be certain of what the cow is eating is to contact the company.

New Zealand has an almost exclusive pasture diet for its cows. Unsalted Anchor Butter from New Zealand is 100 percent grass-fed, fairly affordable, and it has a nice color to it. Apparently some Walmart stores carry it, it can be special ordered from many grocery stores, and it is found online.

You may find some smaller brands of grass-fed butters that have a nice yellow color available in your area. These are also a tasty option. For people who are concerned about the fact that the butter is pasteurized, you can convert the butter into ghee. My favorite ghee is available at traditionafoods.org. If you are not pleased with your level of strengthening of your alveolar bone and periodontal ligament; i.e., your teeth still feel loose when consuming pasteurized butters, then you will need to try a more potent form of activator X/"K2," such as the X-Factor gold butter concentrate.

Fish eggs can be obtained from preservative-free caviar, Japanese food markets, and seasonally from good fish merchants. When I lived in Santa Cruz, California, the local fish warehouse would discard the entire fish carcasses of locally caught fish after removing the fillets. Many of the discarded fish were filled with eggs. At traditionalfoods.org, I plan to have dried fish eggs available for purchase at some point.

We do not just need vitamins to cure gum disease, but we also need minerals that synergize with the vitamins in our diet.

Summary for Vitamins to Cure Gum Disease Naturally

The purpose with this level of detail is so that you can refer back to these lists to help you hone in on exactly what foods can be of the most benefit to you for healing gum disease naturally. This list below summarizes some of the key vitamins and what foods they are in.

- ☐ Seventy percent of Dr. Price's patients with dental problems tested having borderline or low vitamin A. Vitamin A is found exclusively in animal foods such as fermented cod liver oil, liver, goat cheese, butter or ghee, egg yolk, whole milk, and other foods.
- ☐ B1 deficiency can result in hypersensitivity and erosion of the soft tissues in the mouth. Vitamin B1 is found in pork, macadamia nuts, pine nuts, and sunflower seeds, trout, salmon and tuna, and other foods.
- ☐ A B2-deficient diet can create mouth lesions and gingivitis. Vitamin B2 is found in lamb, beef, pork, chicken, turkey liver, mackerel, and almonds.
- ☐ Vitamin B3 deficiency can result in inflammation, redness, soreness, and irritation of the mouth.[58] Vitamin B3 is found in chicken, tuna, sturgeon, beef liver, mackerel, salmon, swordfish, pork meat, and other foods.
- ☐ Folate deficiency has been correlated with gum disease. Vitamin B9 is found in chicken, turkey, duck liver, chicken / turkey giblets, black or mung beans, chickpeas, lentils, and other foods.
- ☐ Studies have connected anemia and periodontal disease with vitamin B12 deficiencies. Vitamin B12 is found in clams, lamb, turkey, beef, pork and chicken liver, oysters, mussels, mackerel, herring, crab, and other foods.
- ☐ The importance of vitamin C to the gingival and alveolar bone has been amply demonstrated in human and animal experiments. Vitamin C is found in high levels in organic acerola powder, and is also found in guava, papaya, parsley, kiwi, oranges, camu camu, and other foods.
- ☐ **Vitamin D is absolutely crucial for healing gum disease**. Diets deficient in vitamins A and D lead to advanced periodontal disease. Vitamin D is necessary to utilize calcium, phosphorus, and other trace minerals. Vitamin D is found in fermented cod liver oil, X-Factor Gold™ high vitamin butter oil, wild tilapia, salmon, herring, pastured duck eggs, and other foods.
- ☐ Activator X/"K2" is a substance not adequately provided for in a typical diet. It leads to the normalization of the blood calcium and phosphorus ratios, which dramatically aids in the healing and prevention of gum disease. Activator X/"K2" synergizes with vitamin D for profound tooth and alveolar bone remineralization. Activator X/"K2" is most easily found in grass-fed yellow butter and fish eggs. It is likely in bone marrow as well.
- ☐ It is recommended that cod liver oil be taken in combination with butter to optimize the nutrients.

5 Restoring Lost Minerals to Cure Gum Disease

Healing gum disease requires restoring adequate levels of vitamins and minerals to our diet from sources that our body can recognize and metabolize—whole foods. Calcium is the most important mineral needed by far to reverse gum disease.

Calcium Stops Gum Disease

Based on the work of Drs. Hawkins and Page, we learned that when the loss of calcium exceeds the body's requirement for this mineral, there could be disintegration and eventual destruction of the alveolar process that supports the teeth.

Calcium Protects Against Alveolar Bone Loss

Dr. Hawkins' forgotten remedy for gum disease was a high calcium diet, combined with alkalizing foods and a moderation of high phosphorous foods (red meats and grains). As was discussed in chapter three, low blood calcium directly correlates with severe periodontal disease. Other literature also shows direct correlations with low calcium intake, imbalanced calcium to phosphorus ratio, and severe periodontal bone loss.[1] The less calcium one eats, the more severe the periodontal disease.[2] The calcium and phosphorus ratio in the blood is maintained by an adequate calcium intake along with the ability to metabolize calcium, which requires fat-soluble vitamins, a balanced glandular system, trace minerals, and a healthy digestive system.

Dairy Products Help Cure Gum Disease

A more recent study shows an inverse relationship between periodontal disease and dairy consumption.[3] The more dairy products people consumed, the lower the prevalence of periodontal disease.[4]

Pasteurization Damages Milk

Many people have learned from an unpleasant experience that pasteurized milk makes them sick or congested and as a result they avoid it. This is rarely due to the commonly blamed lactose intolerance; rather, it is most often due to *pasteurization* and grain-fed milk intolerance. Probably pasteurization's worst offense is that it makes an important portion of the calcium contained in raw milk non-absorbable. Pasteurization also destroys probiotics, which have been shown to be beneficial for periodontal disease.[5] Pasteurization was introduced as an attempt to neutralize (kill) pathogens found in dirty milk from filthy and inhumane "distillery dairies" in the mid 1800s.[6] It was never intended for clean milk from healthy animals on pasture.

In order to absorb calcium from milk, we need the enzyme phosphatase, which is naturally present in raw milk. High temperature pasteurization typically heats milk to 165 degrees or more, and thereby destroys phosphatase.[7] Significant portions of other vitamins are lost in the pasteurization process as well, such as vitamin C. Typically the conventionally produced milk that most people drink contains fecal matter, blood, and pus. Commercial milk must be pasteurized to render it even drinkable. Pasteurization cooks this material. It is not surprising that significant portions of the population are allergic to this toxic soup.

Because pasteurization damages the probiotic content of raw milk, pathogenic organisms associated with disease can easily grow unchecked in pasteurized milk. When the probiotic organisms are destroyed, pasteurized milk lacks its own protective mechanism against harboring toxins that make people sick. In 2007, three people died from drinking pasteurized milk in Massachusetts. Many times when people get sick from milk it is assumed that the milk was not pasteurized properly. Again, as with the diseases of tooth decay or gum disease, bacteria are always blamed. Toxic foods, sick animals, and residues of antibiotics and growth hormones are never considered to be the cause of poisoning from pasteurized milk. Even worse, because milk was pasteurized, doctors will automatically eliminate it as a likely source of causing a particular illness. As a result, sickness caused by pasteurized milk is vastly under reported, while sickness claimed to be caused by raw milk is vastly over reported. With clean hygienic milking standards, healthy raw milk from grass-fed animals is far safer than pasteurized milk from confined animals in concentrated dairy operations.[8]

Homogenized cow's milk renders many nutrients in the milk unusable to the body because the process breaks apart the milk fats' cellular structure. It does so by forcing milk at high pressure through extremely small holes which rupture the wall of fat cells, preventing the fat from rising to the surface of the milk as it would do

Pasteurized Milk and Gum Disease

While cats naturally thrive on raw milk, cats drinking pasteurized milk over time develop gum disease and arthritis. Cats fed pasteurized milk eventually suffer bone loss in their jaws and lose all their teeth.[9]

naturally. Do not drink homogenized milk. Many commercial ice creams are made with homogenized milk to give it a creamier texture.

Commercial dairy animals are injected with rBGH (recombinant bovine growth hormone), and they are fed genetically modified grains, which are not a part of their natural diet. Avoid non-organic dairy foods.

Raw Grass-fed Milk

Consuming pasteurized commercial milk raises the level of non-absorbable calcium in one's diet.[10] However, we've all heard that milk is a good source of calcium. That would be true of raw milk, which is not pasteurized. Milk is spoken of reverentially in the bible as pure and sacred nourishment, and ancient societies correlated milk with health, abundance, and fertility. It is a delicious and healthful gift from the animals. High quality raw milk will substantially contribute to the health and well-being of you and your children. Milk is very high in calcium and phosphorus, which we know now we need for strong teeth and strong alveolar bones. When pastured (not to be confused with pasteurizing), cows eat grass in the time of rapid growth after the rains of early summer and autumn, so there will be moderate amounts of bone hardening activator X/"K2" in the milk.

Before the recent invention of refrigerators, milk was consumed either immediately after milking, known as sweet milk, or it naturally began to sour and was transformed with cultures into cheese and fermented milk like yogurt. Probiotics are vital to our health, support good digestion, and aid in periodontal health.[11] Many forms of soured milk are excellent for obtaining beneficial and vitamin-creating bacteria. Having healthy gums is a result of more than just eating well; it is about absorbing the nutrients in food well. An essential aspect of nutrient absorption is having a diet rich in probiotic, live foods. In addition to a wide spectrum of probiotic bacteria, different forms of soured milk including yogurt contain highly absorbable forms of calcium. Soured milk is also low in milk sugar, known as lactose. A more recent study shows that people who consume more fermented dairy products (like yogurt) had less severe periodontal disease than those who did not.[12]

People in excellent health consume milk in many different forms such as buttermilk, clabber, cottage cheese, kefir, and yogurt. Several ancient Ayurvedic texts describe using milk—yes, raw, grass-fed milk—as a cure for literally hundreds of ailments. The most particularly healing milk to the body was identified as buttermilk. Since all milk was cultured in those days (the refrigerator was not yet invented), this would of course be non-pasteurized cultured buttermilk. Part of milk's healing power lies in its nutrient density and the ease with which our body can digest it.

Let's review some of the life-affirming, mostly cultured, varieties of raw milk:

Clabber is a pleasantly soured yogurt-like milk product produced by allowing milk to sit out in a jar at room temperature.

Kefir (pronounced *keh-FEER*) is produced when milk is cultured with kefir "grains," or organisms. The kefir grains are a symbiotic matrix colony of bacteria and yeast that resemble a piece of cauliflower. Kefir grains can be obtained online, or from friends making kefir at home. At room temperature, the kefir grains consume milk sugars and transform raw milk into a potent, nutrient-rich, cultured beverage. It can be drunk plain or in smoothies. Kefir culture seeds our intestines with milk-digesting bacteria and aids in cleansing and detoxification of the body. Regular consumption of kefir will increase your vitality and longevity by filling you up with more than sixty beneficial yeasts and bacteria, not to mention the highly digestible forms of calcium and other minerals found in kefir milk.

Whey is the light yellowish liquid that remains when milk solids are removed from cultured milk. You may have seen it on the top (or at the bottom) of your yogurt container. After milk sours, the liquid portion of the milk can be separated from the solids, leaving you with curds and whey. Whey is an ancient health remedy because of its ease of digestion along with its vast probiotic contents. Whey can be obtained from yogurt if you do not have access to raw milk.

Buttermilk is the liquid that is left over from the process of churning butter. It has a refreshing sweet and sour taste, and will aid your overall health.

Room temperature milk can be easier to digest than milk fresh out of the refrigerator. Consider warming your milk to room temperature.

Milk Can Be Mislabeled

Some milk laws are backward these days. Milk laws are controlled at the state level, so the law may be different in your state. Dairy products that are sold in larger chain stores labeled as kefir, buttermilk, cottage cheese, or cream cheese are in fact counterfeit. Because of these laws, real kefir, real buttermilk, and real cream cheese are banned from our stores. Instead, the products you see have a specific strain of culture added to the milk or cream to create these products. The natural, old-fashioned way to make these products is through fermentation without adding enzymes. Store products, besides yogurt, do not benefit from the natural culturing process and are dramatically inferior. Usually the taste is completely different from what the real food, generally not available in stores, actually tastes like. Equally, the health benefits from the store-bought products will not be the same as those made from honest, fresh raw milk.

The problem with store-bought dairy is not just in the culturing process, but also in the quality of the original milk used. Some milk products labeled as organic may not come from cows that are raised completely on their natural diet. Instead of being on grass, they are fed organic grains and other fodder, which is not natural to a cow's diet. The result of this large scale, profit-driven production is that the grain-fed milk lacks wholesome life-sustaining nutrients. In general, people do not do well on grain-fed milk; it is too sweet and nutrient deficient. Unless clearly labeled as grass-fed, you can assume that store-bought milk is completely grain-fed, even the organic varieties. If we see a new product in the store we are interested in, we call the farm to learn what conditions the dairy animal was raised under. Although the ideal of organic milk is that it comes from pasture-fed, free ranging cows, the reality is that many larger dairies selling organic milk in grocery stores do not meet these optimal standards.

Obtaining Raw Milk

Due to laws that assault our personal freedoms, liberty, and the right to choose guaranteed by state and the U.S. Constitution, raw milk can be difficult to obtain. In many states raw milk is harder to get than hard liquor, cigarettes, guns, marijuana, and prescription drugs that have known dangerous side effects. The facetious term for raw milk in locales where it is illegal to be sold to the public is "moo-shine."

realmilk.com - One easy way to find raw milk in your vicinity.

westonaprice.org - Get involved with and contact your local Weston A. Price Foundation chapter leader. Many times they can direct you to lesser known cow-share programs and legal direct-from-the-farmer dairy products.

Whole Foods Market® has a very nice artisan cheese section with many raw milk cheeses. You can tell if a cheese is grass-fed typically by how pungent it is. Grain-fed cheese has a bland or "normal" milk flavor. Grass-fed cheese is flavorful, usually pungent, and sometimes contains hints of a grassy flavor. In cities or more affluent areas, you can often find cheese mongers who will have several varieties of grass-fed raw cheeses, many of which are imported from Europe. If you like cheese, do yourself a favor and try some new varieties.

Dairy Sensitivities

Many people are told that they cannot digest dairy foods, or experience negative effects from pasteurized milk. Yet for a majority of people these negative effects do not occur when they drink raw, grass-fed milk. This is because raw, grass-fed milk is a completely different product from pasteurized confinement dairy milk. If raw cow's milk does not work for you, but you still want to consume dairy, then I highly recommend starting with soured milk in the form of kefir or yogurt. Also do not be afraid to try milk from other animals such as sheep, goat, camel, or mare's milk. Some milk consumers who cannot tolerate fluid milk find that they have no problems with really good cheese. Over a period of months, consuming real kefir will restore most people's ability to drink raw milk. If you are unable to tolerate dairy products, then usually it is a sign that your digestive system is not working properly. Consider strategies, such as those that will be discussed in chapter seven, to restore the full functioning of your digestive system so that you can enjoy a wider range of calcium-rich foods.

The goal for calcium consumption for a healthy adult is somewhere between 1-1½ grams of calcium per day. For acute oral conditions, many people will temporarily benefit from a higher dose of absorbable calcium, which I estimate to be from 1.6-2.2 grams.

Four cups (one quart) of milk provides about one gram of calcium and one gram of phosphorus per day. This is a significant portion of your daily requirements of the minerals you need for healthy teeth and a healthy jawbone. As a note, cream or cream cheese contains the fat portion of the milk, which has very little calcium, but plenty of fat-soluble vitamins needed to absorb the calcium.

Calcium Content in Foods

RDI 1,000-1,200 mg/day
(Dr. Weston Price recommended 1,500 mg/day)

Food	**Calcium in Milligrams**
Traditional Foods Whole Bone Calcium – ½ teaspoon	720 mg
Hard / Soft cheeses – 2 ounces	404 mg
Traditional Foods Bone Marrow Calcium – 1 teaspoon	400 mg
Canned sardines with bones – 1 can 3.75 ounces	351 mg
Goat milk – 1 cup	327 mg
Yogurt, whole milk – 1 cup	296 mg
Canned salmon with bones – 3.5 ounces	277 mg
Whole milk – 1 cup	276 mg
Cooked collard greens – 1 cup	266 mg
Cooked Tahitian taro root – 1 cup	204 mg
Cooked kale – 1 cup	171 mg
Cooked beet greens – 1 cup	164 mg
Cooked dandelion greens – 1 cup	147 mg
Cooked broccoli – 2 cups	120 mg
Traditional corn tortillas – 3 at 4.2 ounces	120+ mg
Cooked scallops – 3.5 ounces	115 mg
Cooked white beans – ½ cup	113 mg
Herring – 3 ounces	90 mg
Sesame seeds – 1 tablespoon	89 mg
Heavy cream – ½ cup	78 mg
Cottage cheese – ½ cup	69 mg
Tahini roasted – 1 tablespoon	64 mg
Halibut – 3 ounces	50 mg
Cooked pinto beans – ½ cup	45 mg
Sweet potato, one medium	40 mg
Shrimp – 3 ounces	33 mg
Salmon without bones – 3.5 ounces	28 mg

Short Term Dairy Intake per Day for Acute Imbalances People deficient in calcium will need 1,600-2,200 mg of calcium per day.
6-8 cups of raw dairy per day (cow, goat, sheep, etc.) Make sure to regularly include any or all of these probiotic cultured milk products: kefir, yogurt, clabber, whey, and/or buttermilk or
6-10 ounces of (preferably) raw cheese per day (cow, goat, sheep, etc.) or
½-1½ teaspoons of Grass-fed Whole Bone Calcium matrix or
1.5-3 teaspoons of Grass-fed Bone Marrow Calcium

For best results, mix and match your calcium sources. If possible, include some raw fluid milk like yogurt or kefir, some raw or artisanally produced cheese, and some calcium from bones such as from chewing on the well-cooked ends of chicken bones.

Bone supplements that can help are *Whole Bone Calcium* which is freeze-dried, grass-fed beef bone, and *Bone, Marrow, and Cartilage* which is grass-fed veal bone including the nutrient-dense marrow and cartilage. Both are available from traditionalfoods.org.

If your calcium levels are adequate, or you do not find yourself in an urgent condition, then the adequate calcium intake would average from around 1.2g-1.5g per day. **Make sure to listen to your body and get help if necessary to fine tune your calcium needs. These figures are just estimates; everyone is different.**

Maintenance Food-Based Calcium Dose 1,200mg-1,500mg daily

Non-Dairy Calcium Alternatives

To obtain adequate dietary calcium without using dairy foods, dentist Melvin Page recommended eating salmon, oysters, clams, shrimp, other sea foods, broccoli, beet greens, nuts, beans, cauliflower, figs, and olives.[13] Green vegetables that are very high in calcium come from the brassica family and include broccoli, kale, bok choy, cabbage, mustard, and turnip greens. Other sources of calcium could be taro root and herbs. To maximize calcium absorption, eat these vegetables with plenty of butter or ghee (or other fat if you cannot tolerate any dairy). Those who avoid dairy will do best having some type of naturally-occurring bone calcium. Often, people do not absorb calcium well from vegetable sources. Even with the following supplement and diary-free example, adequate calcium is only obtained by adding sardines with the bones to the menu. Therefore, if you do not consume dairy products at all, make sure to add some type of bone product to your diet.

Here is one example of how it would be done:

- 1 entire can of sardines with bones, 351 mg
- 2 cups of cooked collard greens, 532 mg (may not be absorbed well unless butter or other fats/oils are eaten with it)
- 2 cups of cooked kale, 342 mg (consume with some fat like butter)

Total – 1,225 milligrams of calcium

Bone Consumption

In some traditional diets, people like to gnaw, chew, and suck on bones for a long period of time. Of course, not all bones are edible or can be broken down, but many can. The easiest way to consume bones is with a well-cooked chicken soup. At home we use the Kuhn Rikon pressure cooker to speedily make our soups. Both a traditional long cooking time and pressure-cooking chicken bones will break down the joint ends of the bones. The ends of the chicken bones should dissolve or crunch easily when fully cooked. Consider eating the soft portions of them, including the cartilage, as they are rich in calcium and marrow, as well as tasty. Bone broth is not rich in calcium, contrary to what you might expect, but it is rich in collagen from the cartilaginous portions of bones, which is also important for strengthening your jawbone and teeth.

The traditional practice of roasting fish bones or chewing on certain fish bones is another way calcium was traditionally obtained in the diet. For example, the cartilaginous bones in the head of the salmon can be sucked on and broken down. If this is your first time doing this, proceed with care; don't swallow any bones whole. Parts of the bone will break down if chewed on. Fish heads also often have easily chewed round chunks of calcium at certain places. I have also put together two food-based calcium supplements made from bones to support getting one's daily calcium needs. They are available at traditionalfoods.org.

Calcium Supplements

Many, but not all, calcium supplements contain forms of calcium that are not recognized by your body. Non-absorbable calcium can raise blood calcium levels in an unhealthy way, which can lead to excess calculus deposits. Use extra care when selecting your calcium supplements.

Eggshells can also be an alternative source of calcium.

1. Clean eggshells can be thoroughly air-dried and powdered in a coffee or spice grinder.
2. Mix one dozen powdered eggshells with 2 cups of apple cider vinegar (use a large container as it will foam).

It can be left at room temperature, and you can use two or more tablespoons per day of the liquid. It can be difficult to digest the plain ground up eggshells not soaked in vinegar.

Trace Minerals for Healing Gum Disease and Balancing Body Chemistry

Dr. Page found that without trace minerals, our glandular system falls out of balance. When our glands become imbalanced, so do our calcium and phosphorous ratios. By replacing trace minerals, in many instances the assimilation of and utilization of calcium and phosphorus significantly increases.[14]

Minerals feed our glands and control the intricate fluid systems of our body.[15] When dietary trace minerals are replaced, the glandular system can start to regulate itself.

Powdered sea kelp is so essential to balancing our glands, that Dr. Page started his own company selling kelp powder. He would prescribe five or six five-grain tablets of kelp to his patients per day, which equates to 1.6–1.9 grams of kelp. Roughly speaking, this is a third to a half teaspoon of kelp powder per day. Kelp powder is by far one of the most effective and affordable mineral and trace mineral supplements available. Consuming kelp powder regularly is an excellent way to remineralize your body.

Iodine is a key element needed for health as it activates and stabilizes the endocrine glands and is responsible for normal nerve impulses. Iodine also supports mental activity and intellect, as well as the proper metabolism of calcium, phosphorus, and carbohydrates.

Thyroid problems, especially hypothyroid conditions, may negatively affect gum health.[16] We need healthy thyroid and parathyroid function to metabolize calcium and maintain our metabolism. As discussed in chapter three, when our minerals are out of balance, so too are our glands. Common environmental and food toxins like fluoride, chlorine, and bromide all interfere with iodine uptake, causing relative deficiencies. In the past, less iodine would have been sufficient to maintain health, but more is needed today in the presence of toxins to remain healthy and balanced. Iodine is likely an important micronutrient for healing tooth and gum problems.

There is quite a debate on how much iodine is healthy to take.[17] A recent literature review shows that in the seaweed-rich diet of Japan, the average person consumes 1,000 to 3,000 mcg (1-3 mg) of iodine per day.[18] Kelp seems to be by far the most iodine-rich source of seaweed. The U.S. Government RDI for iodine is 150mcg (0.15mg). So you should be aware that taking the suggested amount of kelp might take you above the Government's "upper limit" of iodine, which is set at 1,100 mcg. To make it easier for you to get the best quality kelp powder available, I have organic kelp powder available at traditionalfoods.org.

Kelp Powder Dosage for Minerals
¼-½ teaspoon of kelp powder per day, 4-6 days per week

Important notes: Kelp contains trace elements and metals naturally occurring in the ocean in small amounts. Some people may need to take smaller doses of kelp. As always, use your best judgment and seek professional help when necessary to determine if kelp powder is right for you, and how much to take.

Zinc for Healing Gum Tissues

Zinc likely plays a very important role in periodontal disease.[19] A decrease of zinc in the body can lead to increased permeability of bacteria (lowered host defense) associated with gingivitis.[20] In a series of eighty periodontal patients with severe gum disease, high blood copper was found to directly relate with periodontal disease.[21] Copper toxicity is likely to occur in women who take birth control pills or who use an IUD, and copper and zinc imbalances are common in vegans and vegetarians.[22] High blood copper is an increasingly common problem because of xenoestrogen (such as in plastics and pesticides) and phytoestrogen (soy) exposure.

Zinc helps the body restore its acid / alkaline balance and helps people recover from periodontal disease. Low zinc levels are also a big risk factor in male infertility.[23]

Foods High in Zinc

RDI 8-11 mg

Food	Zinc in Milligrams
Oysters – 6 raw	30-76 mg
Red meat of various types – 3.5 ounces	8 mg
Crab and lobster / various types – 3.5 ounces	4-5 mg
Oyster Power supplement – 4 capsules	3 mg

Eating oysters a few times a week is an amazingly healthy practice, which will over the course of a week give you an average of 14-20 milligrams of zinc per day.

Suggested Zinc Intake
6 oysters 2-4 times per week or 4-12 capsules of powdered oysters 2-4 times per week

Low Budget: For those on a restricted budget, buying pre-shucked oysters in a jar will provide the most oyster meat for the least amount of money.

Optimal: Fresh oysters are an absolutely amazing and life-giving food—an excellent fishmonger or seafood restaurant should offer their oysters fresh-shucked when you order. We bought an oyster knife and learned how to do it ourselves—they are usually not too hard to shuck with a little practice.

Alternative: For those who cannot get good oysters or who do not want to eat them, zinc in its naturally occurring form is available in Oyster Power, which is pure, low-temperature dried oysters. Four to sixteen capsules per day will really boost your zinc level for enhanced energy and vitality. The average to support gum health would be six to eight capsules of Oyster Power. It is available at: traditionalfoods.org.

Non-Oyster Sources of Zinc: I recommend zinc from oysters and secondarily from red meat and other shellfish. Truly naturally-occurring zinc is in the exact form that nature intended for humans to consume it, and it contains the perfect amount of co-factors such as manganese, copper, and selenium. Synthetic zinc supplements can be problematic because one can easily take too much, and other trace minerals can fall out of balance because they are not mixed with zinc in a whole foods matrix. If you choose to use synthetic zinc, do so with caution.

Magnesium

There is very little direct evidence relating gum disease to magnesium. However a low blood level of magnesium may contribute to a low blood level of calcium.[24]

Foods High in Magnesium

RDI 320-420 mg

Food	Magnesium in Milligrams
Mackerel, salmon, halibut, pollock – 3.5 ounces	86-120 mg
Brazil nuts – 6	106 mg
Swiss chard – ½ cup	75 mg
Corn tortillas – 4 tortillas – 3.5 ounces	72 mg
Sesame seed butter, sunflower seed butter – 1 tablespoon	56-59 mg
Pine nuts – 1 ounce	42 mg

It is actually difficult for most Americans to meet the daily minimum requirement of 320 mg of magnesium for women and 420 mg for men from food. For this reason, consider trying a fun and soothing way to obtain this mineral from magnesium bath flakes that come from the Zechstein ancient sea bed in the Netherlands. Taking a magnesium bath two to four times a week or using magnesium topical "oil" two to four times per week seems like a safe way to add a magnesium boost to your system. The bath flakes and "oil" are also conveniently available at traditionalfoods.org.

Selenium

I could not find direct correlations between selenium and periodontal disease. Nevertheless it might be useful to have adequate selenium in your diet. Brazil nuts are very high in selenium, and so is most seafood including oysters, squid, and fish of various sorts, and of course, liver.

Iron

I also could not find direct correlations between iron and gum disease; however, iron is an important mineral. Foods high in iron are already on our food lists and include animal livers and mollusks such as clams, mussels, and oysters.

Salt for Gum Health

Dr. Hawkins found that many people with Type 1 gum disease had high potassium levels and poor salt retention. Having enough or plenty of salt will help balance this. Commercial, highly refined table salt is irritating to the body. Real salt plays a key role in digestion and many people with gum disease do not have healthy digestive systems. Salt contains chloride, which is an important ingredient needed for hydrochloric acid production, therefore having enough salt in our diet will support healthy digestion. Low salt diets are directly correlated with diabetes.[25] This should be of particular interest to us because diabetes is directly connected with gum disease. Salt is necessary for the electrical system of our body. Historically, the average daily consumption worldwide of salt is 1.5 to 3 teaspoons.[26]

Suggested Salt Intake
1+ teaspoons per day

Important notes about salt: Some foods naturally have salt, so consider that in your daily salt intake. I recommend sun dried sea salt from France. Celtic Salt is one such brand available at many natural food stores. For your convenience you can buy excellent salt with free shipping at: traditionalfoods.org.

Good Soup Helps Heal Your Gums

Collagen is a major building block of the periodontium.[27] In chapter three I mentioned that the alveolar bone, which deteriorates in the course of gum disease, is about 28 percent collagen. It is therefore sensible to support the reconstruction and health of our bones by consuming a food that will help build our own collagen. This food is gelatin, which is derived from collagen.

There's nothing like delicious, gelatin-rich soup to warm our insides on a cold day. Homemade broths are an important remedy for gum disease. Broth from nourishing soup is made by boiling cartilage-rich bones of chicken, beef, fish, and so on. Good broth is rich in gelatin, and when refrigerated it will gel. Excellent gravy can be made with beef, lamb, or turkey broth.

Gelatin can help heal and rebuild the digestive tract. It enhances protein absorption when consumed with meals. Aloe vera and slippery elm bark gruel can also aid in soothing the intestines. The best bone broth for gum disease reversal is broth made from the carcasses of wild fish. The carcass ideally should have the head, and if it has the organs—even better. This broth is especially potent and rich in minerals. *Instructions for fish broth can be found at:* **curegumdisease.com/broth**. Healthy cultures around the world know the value of soup made with fish heads. The meat, eyes, and brain from the fish are all eaten, as they are rich in minerals and fat-soluble vitamins.

Suggested Broth Consumption
1-2 cups of broth per day, 4-6 days per week. Consume it as a tea, in soups, in stews, or as gravy

Alternatives to Making Soup

Gelatin is collagen that has extracted from skin, bones, and connective tissues of animals and been broken down. It occurs naturally in the diet if you consume cartilaginous pieces of animal foods and their skin.

- □ ½ -1 teaspoon per day of *bone, marrow, and cartilage*
- □ 1 teaspoon per day of gelatin powder (makes 1 cup of gelatin when mixed with water)

Both are conveniently available at traditionalfoods.org.

Coconut Oil for Thyroid Health

Coconut oil increases metabolic rate and can normalize thyroid function.[28] Since a healthy thyroid function is needed for optimal calcium metabolism, I believe most readers would benefit from consuming one to three teaspoons of coconut oil per day, four to six days per week.

Summary of Chapters Four and Five, Restoring Lost Vitamin and Minerals:

- Healing gum disease requires vitamins A, B, C, D, and Activator X (K2).
- Liver is the best source of vitamin A and the B vitamins. B vitamins are essential for gum health.
- Vitamin C is essential to healthy gum tissues and connective tissue, and many cases of gum disease have a likely component of sub-acute vitamin deficiency.
- Cod liver oil taken with butter is extremely effective in mineralizing tissues and making loose teeth stronger due to its high vitamin A and D and activator X contents.
- Raw dairy products, or food-based calcium supplements, are essential to achieving adequate calcium intake. Many people digest fermented forms of raw dairy better than just fresh raw milk.
- Kelp powder will support overall glandular function and assist with the utilization and metabolism of food, as well as balancing blood chemistry.

6 Toxic Modern Foods and Environmental Stresses That Cause and Contribute to Gum Disease

Dr. Weston Price showed the dramatic negative impact that modern, industrially processed foods can have on our bodies. Clearly, in order to obtain a healthy body, including healthy gums, we need to avoid such foods.

The Characteristics of a Disease-Forming Diet

Neither the dental industry nor universities have found the true cause of gum disease, nor have they been able to describe how to stop it. They do not know how to heal diseases, because they themselves are not healthy. Thus, listening to conventional dietary advice will lead us down the same path to the same poor health as those who have blazed this path.

Consider this example from Dr. Price:

> *The cook on the government boat was an aboriginal Australian from Northern Australia. He had been trained on a military craft as a dietitian. Nearly all his teeth were lost. It is of interest that while the native Aborigines had relatively perfect teeth, this man who was a trained dietitian for the whites had lost nearly all his teeth from tooth decay and pyorrhea.*[1]

I encourage you to think for yourself when it comes to what is healthy. Much of the dietary advice we hear today is seeded by corporate nefarious intentions to entice us to eat foods that are robust profit drivers for the industry, yet are counterfeit nutrition and harmful to us. If you are not already committed to real foods and healthy eating, this chapter may seem daunting to you. If you are willing to seriously seek only the best nutrition available, then this chapter will help you fine tune your diet to avoid any foods that might be contributing to your gum disease.

Avoid Toxic Grains and Flour

I love grains and eat them regularly. If consumed without any preparation, however, grains can deplete your body of minerals. If consumed once they are properly prepared, grains can be a nourishing food.

One recipe for creating gum disease is a diet high in meat and grains and low in calcium from dairy products. A diet that heavily favors meat and grains and is also low in calcium is disproportionately high in phosphorus and can contribute to a calcium/phosphorus imbalance in the body that may lead to gum disease.

William Lorentz, professor of dentistry, observed the connection between gum disease and diet in the 1930s, finding that patients afflicted with gum disease heavily consumed wheat flour products, such as bread, biscuits, pancakes, doughnuts, pastries, and cereals, and only lightly consumed foods rich in needed minerals. His analysis after examining hundreds of patients with gum disease revealed that patients with periodontal disease heavily consumed wheat.[2] Dr. Price reported that the principal source of calories in modern disease-promoting diets came from white flour. The problem with too much wheat is that it can replace more nutrient-dense foods in the diet. I strongly suggest eliminating all processed white flour foods from your diet.

Nearly every packaged, industrially processed product that contains grain should be eliminated from the diet. **Also avoid sprouted whole grain products and gluten-free foods made with brown rice.**

These industrially made products often contain additives such as anti-caking agents, stabilizers, leavening agents, or acidifiers such as tricalcium phosphate, trimagnesium phosphate, disodium phosphate, and dipotassium phosphate. Many times these chemicals are not even listed on labels. These additives are another reason to avoid commercially produced foods.[3]

These days there are organic varieties of almost every one of the wheat products listed on the next page. Some people will tolerate them while others will not. I have found that the best way to consume wheat in the long run is for the products to be made from unbleached (sifted) organic flour that has been soured (fermented). If you do choose to consume other organic wheat products and find that you continue to suffer from tooth decay or gum disease, then the wheat, regardless of its form, may be a significant culprit. Do watch out for whole grain varieties of these

Foods That Are Often Made with White Flour That Can Wreck Your Gums

crackers	muffins	pasta
cookies	biscuits	pizza
doughnuts	pastries	pancakes
pies	white flour tortillas	waffles
breakfast cereals	bagels	croissants
granola	noodles	toaster tarts

foods as well since phytic acid, which is concentrated in the bran and germ, can cause nutrient losses and demineralization of the alveolar bone and teeth.

Phytic Acid and Your Oral Health

Phytic acid is the principal storage form of phosphorus in many grains, especially the bran portion of grains and other seeds. It is found in significant amounts in grains, nuts, beans, seeds, and some tubers. Phytic acid contains the mineral phosphorus tightly bound in a snowflake-like molecule. In humans and animals with one stomach, the phosphorus is not readily absorbable by normal digestion. In addition to blocking dietary phosphorus availability, the "arms" of the phytic acid molecule readily bind with (chelate) other minerals, such as calcium, magnesium, iron, and zinc, making them unavailable as well.

Adding vitamin C to the diet can significantly counteract phytic acid's iron absorption blocking effect.[4] This could explain why symptoms of scurvy, such as soft and spongy gums leading to tooth loss, are the result of both a lack of vitamin C and a heavy whole grain diet of hardtack.

Phytic acid strongly blocks mineral absorption in adults.[5] It not only uses up the minerals in our body, but also inhibits the enzymes we need to break down our food. Phytic acid furthermore inhibits pepsin,[6] which is needed for the breakdown of proteins in the stomach: amylase, which starts the breakdown of starch into sugar in the mouth,[7] and trypsin, needed for protein digestion in the small intestine.[8] The concentration of and types of enzyme inhibitors vary considerably among different types of grains.[9] Grains contain tannins, which can depress growth, decrease iron absorption, and damage the mucosal lining of the gastrointestinal tract. Grains also contain saponins, which can inhibit growth.[10]

Traditional groups did not avoid gluten-containing foods, and they certainly did not go to stores to buy gluten-free cookies. Rather they carefully harvested, stored, and prepared grains to ensure these foods would promote health and vitality. Today, grains have become the bane of many people's health, leading some to steer clear of grains, or even to avoid carbohydrate foods altogether.

Indigenous peoples who valued grains as a dietary staple consistently used ingenious preparation methods to remove their anti-nutritional factors. Such methods included souring or fermenting, soaking with lye or lime salts, and removing the bran and other fibrous parts of various grains.

Bran is high in insoluble fiber that your body cannot digest. Indigenous peoples generally remove the bran from grains through sifting or other means and process their foods so they are soft, tasty, and easy to digest. When bran is used as fertilizer, it is first fermented to release its vitamin content. When I was younger, I believed the premise that bran was healthy because it contained many nutrients, so I would force myself to eat bran muffins. Even with the large amount of unhealthy sugar they contained, they tasted terrible. I was not listening to my body when eating those bran muffins. My body did not want to eat bran; it wanted to spit it out. The so-called benefits of consuming the insoluble fiber from bran are unproven. The large bulky material may irritate one's digestive tract.[11] Bran-enriched food, especially bran that is not thoroughly fermented, will have extremely high amounts of demineralizing phytic acid. It is better to focus instead on foods that taste good and are easy to digest and absorb, rather than on foods that the television or government says are good for us but do not provide a sense of well-being.

Phytic Acid Content of Popular Foods

Researchers favor guinea pigs for research on scurvy because guinea pigs, like humans, cannot produce vitamin C on their own. Scurvy is of particular interest to us because of the severe tooth and gum problems that result from the condition.[12] And the problem is not limited to vitamin C. Scurvy has been induced in guinea pigs by feeding them bran, oats, barley, maize, and soybean flour.[13] In fact, scurvy can kill a guinea pig fed only oats in just twenty-four days.[14] These experiments show the potentially hazardous effects of grain toxins and high whole grain consumption.[15]

Avoid Commercially Made Whole Grain Products

Whole grain products are so heavily marketed as "all natural" and "healthy," that they have become widely accepted as such. Yet the bran and germ of wheat, rye, spelt, kamut, rice, and barley can actually harm us. Recall that sailors on long sea voyages had a diet comprised of mostly hardtack, a simple type of cracker or biscuit made from flour, water, and sometimes salt, which led to loose teeth and bleeding gums.

Yeasted whole grain breads have 40–80 percent of their phytic acid intact in the finished product.[16] If a yeasted bread is made with unbleached organic white flour, however, it will not contain much phytic acid, as the bran has been removed. I have heard of several cases of whole grain sourdough bread made from spelt that contributed to severe tooth decay. This is because fermentation, while good at reducing phytic acid, does not neutralize all the grain toxins such as lectins in certain varieties of grains. I have also heard of a case of teeth dissolving rapidly from a high consumption of brown rice tortillas. This type of feedback and my own observations have led me to the conclusion that it is best to completely avoid commercially prepared breads, crackers, health food bars, pastas, cereals, and anything else in the grocery store that contains whole grains. Quinoa, buckwheat, amaranth, and teff are exceptions because these are pseudo-cereals and therefore not grains, but care must be taken as to what form you are consuming of those products.

Avoid sprouted grain breads – Another deadly food for teeth and gums is commercially made sprouted grain products from whole grains. The whole grain plant toxins are not sufficiently neutralized by sprouting and these foods can cause significant mineral losses. Nearly all commercially available brands contain soy sprouts.[17] In the case of soy, sprouting in the short term increases its anti-nutritional factors.[18]

Avoid most gluten-free grain products – Today we can eaily buy gluten-free foods, including cookies and other treats. While this has been a boon for many consumers, it is important to remember that gluten-free grains can still contain calcium-leaching anti-nutrients like phytic acid. If you are serious about recovering your health, it is important to avoid industrially processed factory food, even if it is labeled as gluten-free. Gluten-free products typically contain cheap oils, fillers, soy, and other unsavory ingredients.[19]

Many gluten-free products are made with brown rice. Brown rice, or rice bran, is very high in phytic acid and these products should be avoided. Mineral depleting soy flour and other cheaper ingredients are also commonly found in these products. Gluten-free grain products made from white rice, on the other hand, will not have much phytic acid or grain toxins and can be acceptable to use in the context of a mineral-dense diet.

Avoid health food bars – Many contain soy and/or whole grains that are very high in phytates, trypsin inhibitors, and other anti-nutrients. Some also contain high levels of sweeteners that go by various names. Most "health food" bars are so loaded with hard-to-digest whole grains and/or sweeteners that they should be called "tooth decay bars." (Almost all of them are that bad; however, there may be a few exceptions.)

Limit popcorn – Popcorn contains some phytic acid and can also easily get stuck in the teeth and gums. Moderate amounts of popcorn are safe to eat for people who are otherwise healthy.

Bleached Flour vs. Unbleached Flour

Unless labeled as unbleached, white flour has been subjected to benzoyl peroxide or chlorine dioxide to make it appear bright white. Many commercial flours add potassium bromate and are also enriched. Choose unenriched organic unbleached white flour when possible. Flour can go rancid easily, so flour that is freshly ground will be much, much healthier. If not used immediately, freshly ground flour can be stored in the short term in air-tight containers and should be refrigerated or frozen for longer storage.

Food Combining Makes Grains Safer and Healthier

Calcium – When vitamin D is low in the diet, even phytic-acid-free grains can deplete levels of calcium.[20] This gives us an important clue to safe grain consumption—eat foods rich in calcium with your grains. Natives of the Loetschental ate their rye bread with cheese. Calcium will block many negative effects from grains, nuts, and beans. If you consume bread, have it with a large slice of cheese. Enjoy lentils with some yogurt on the side. Know that excess oatmeal consumption can lead to rickets (a disease of imperfect bone formation due to a lack of vitamin D and minerals) but this adverse effect can be limited by calcium.[21]

Vitamin C significantly counteracts the negative effects of grain anti-nutrients. Have vitamin C-rich foods with meals that include grains, nuts, beans, or seeds. Vitamin C is an important part of the program to cure gum disease, so pay close attention to those guidelines especially if you are a heavy grain, nut, bean, seed, or meat eater.

Folate is the naturally occurring form of the nutrient folic acid (which is the synthetic form). Folate may play an important part in working with vitamin C to reduce the anti-nutritional effects of grains. High amounts of folate are found in liver from a variety of animals especially chicken, duck, and goose, as well as in beans, leafy greens, and asparagus. **Vitamin D** – Grain consumption depletes vitamins A and D, but vitamin D in your diet can mitigate that.[22, 23] The more grains we consume, in particular oatmeal or whole grains, the more vitamin D our bodies need. However, there is a limit to the extent that vitamin D will block the negative effect of high consumption of whole grains. That's why even people who are replete in vitamin D can experience periodontal problems. It's also why for those susceptible to gum disease, it is crucial to consume grains with reduced levels of phytic acid and other anti-nutrients found in grains. The combination of low phytic acid grains with vitamin D produced optimal bone growth and protection against rickets in diets that contained grains. To heal the alveolar bone and protect it, optimizing bone growth is essential.

Protein – Traditional nut preparation combines roasted nuts with meat stews. Having protein with grains, nuts, seeds, or beans may reduce some of their anti-nutritional characteristics.

Summary of Basic Grain and Seed Consumption Guidelines

- ☐ Do not eat store-bought products containing whole grains or added bran.
- ☐ Do not eat sprouted whole grain products.
- ☐ Do not consume bleached white flour products and/or non-organic grains.
- ☐ When you consume grains, nuts, seeds, or beans regularly, make sure to include adequate calcium, vitamin C, and vitamin D in your diet.

Healthier Grains

Sourdough bread made from organic unbleached "white" flour will be low in phytic acid. Not all sourdoughs are created equally. The bread should be soured at least sixteen hours and have some sour taste. Ideally, the grain should be freshly ground with a grindstone and have most of the bran and germ removed. The traditional method of preparing bread in the French Alps is with rye flour that has had 25 percent by weight of the resulting flour removed by sifting; this removes nearly all the bran and germ.[24]

White rice does not contain much phytic acid. Strangely, a nutritional comparison of cooked white rice to cooked brown rice shows them to be very comparable in nutrients.[25] It would seem then that the soil quality of where the rice is grown is the bigger factor in its nutritional makeup then whether it is white or brown. It is more sensible to obtain good white rice than it is to consume it whole with its phytate-rich and possibly rancid rice bran. It appears that white jasmine and white basmati rice in health food stores retain a tiny portion of the rice germ because of their brownish color. White rice does not seem to have negative health effects on people the way that white flour does. The ideal way to prepare rice is to use rice that is first aged for one year, then freshly milled to remove half or more of the bran and germ, and finally soaked overnight before cooking. Since most of us cannot do all of this ourselves, our second best options are to choose between high-quality white rice, and partially milled rice. For best results, soak white rice overnight and then discard the water before cooking.

Corn can be an excellent grain, but only when it is organic corn and processed to make it digestible through being nixtamalized with lime salts, or a complex process using lye. Nixtamalization is the process of boiling and soaking dried corn in a highly alkaline, high calcium lime, which is called pickling lime in the U.S. The corn is ideally boiled for at least one hour in the pickling lime, and then soaked for at least twelve hours. Corn tortillas are usually made with nixtamalized corn. I have not found a good masa harina on the market, which is dried nixtamalized corn. The high calcium content of the lime protects against the phytate in the corn germ. Not all brands of corn tortillas are ideal, so make sure to choose organic varieties in order to avoid genetically modified (GMO) corn, which is highly toxic and promotes sterility.

Quinoa, Buckwheat, Amaranth, and Teff

At this time I cannot provide exact instructions for the healthiest methods to prepare these grains. Quinoa does need to be washed several times to eliminate bitterness, since anti-nutrients, such as saponins, reside on the surface of the grain. Buckwheat is best (and tastiest) when sprouted for three to five days, dried, roasted, and boiled, or soaked overnight. Sometime in 2015, I will have free and detailed grain preparation guidelines for most grains available at traditionalfoods.org. Please subscribe to the newsletter to stay informed and updated.

Advanced Grain Guidelines

Traditionally, grains are freshly ground before use. Once the grain is ground, do not use it without first sifting it with a sifter or sieve to remove the bran and germ. Depending on the grain, you'll want to remove 15-25 percent of the entire grain via sifting. Grains that require bran and germ removal to be safe include, but are not limited to, rye, spelt, kamut, barley, oats, and other wheat varieties.

Temporarily Removing Grains

Adults with gum problems would do well to avoid grains for two to three weeks to let their bodies recover and find balance. Chapter eight offers a grain-free diet program. Consider taking a break from grains if:

- You have already adopted a nutrient-dense diet and have achieved some healing success, but not complete success. Perhaps you are experiencing less tooth movement and less bleeding, but still feel inflammation, bleeding, or loose teeth.
- You have been consuming many white flour products or whole grains that were not properly soured. If so, it is possible that your intestinal lining is inflamed. Taking a temporary break from grains will help heal this problem.

After removing grains from the diet for a few weeks, you will be better able to evaluate how they are affecting your body. By introducing properly prepared grains one at a time, you will then be able to determine which grains feel good for you to eat.

Beans and Oral Health

Beans can be delicious foods, but they can also contain many plant toxins. Beans are high in phytic acid and lectins. Lathyrism is a disease attributed to poor people who in times of famine planted and consumed the extremely hardy bean *Lathyrus sativus* (related to the ornamental sweet pea) which is toxic to humans. Soybeans contain many toxins and anti-nutrients and require extensive fermentation to be made safe to consume in modest quantities. Lima beans contain a variety of toxins and yet are consumed in Nigeria as a staple. But, they involve "painstaking processes" to make them safe to eat.[26]

To thoroughly reduce phytates, beans need to be soaked overnight in warm water, geminated for several days, and then soured. Most people will not be able to go to the lengths needed to remove all of the phytic acid in beans and I don't know if the germination process is a traditional method. Soaking beans overnight in a slightly alkaline solution (using a pinch of baking soda for example) and then cooking them eliminates a good portion of phytic acid in smaller beans like lentils. Simply soaking beans overnight may be good enough for most people. Just boiling beans that are not soaked first will not remove a significant amount of phytic acid.

As with grains, different beans have different concentrations of plant toxins, and require different types of preparation methods. The exact details for indigenous cultures' preparation of commonly used beans are unobtainable by me at this time. But we can look at a few examples. In Latin America, beans are often fermented after the cooking process to make a sour porridge called chugo. In India, lentils are typically consumed split. That means the outer layer, the husk (equivalent to the bran in grains), is removed. Lentils without the bran are probably the safest beans to eat. Lentils can be soured into tasty cakes with rice called dosas. Take the same food combining precautions with beans as you would with grains. Eat beans with cheese or yogurt, vitamin D-containing-foods, and vitamin C-rich vegetables.

Bean Suggestions

Basic

- ☐ Soak beans overnight in warm water and cook with kombu (sea vegetable) to soften them and aid digestion.
  - ☐ Beans should be very soft and easy to digest when fully cooked.
  - ☐ Choose smaller sized beans over larger ones.
  - ☐ Eat beans with cheese or some type of dairy product like yogurt.
- ☐ Add spices to the beans to enhance flavor and to increase digestive fire.

Advanced

- ☐ Prepare soured beans in dishes like dosas and chugo.

Cooking beans with kombu (sea kelp) makes the beans more digestible.

Breakfast Cereals and Granola

Store-bought breakfast cereals are unhealthy. Many people unwisely continue to eat cold breakfast cereals because of the sugar-powered high it provides, and ignore the digestive distress that follows. Avoid the rancid and improperly prepared seeds, nuts, and grains found in granolas, quick-rise breads, and extruded breakfast cereals.

Store-bought granola is almost always unhealthy because of its high sugar content and high level of phytic acid from unprocessed oats. The oats are also potentially rancid, or contain mold. The traditional method for storing oats is in air-tight containers before they are pressed or rolled![27] The sugar and flour combination in typical prepared breakfast cereals will cause a rapid rise in blood sugar and thus promote gum disease. Organic store-bought breakfast cereal may not have as many pesticides or additives, but it is not a nourishing food. If you must have cereal I suggest making homemade rice, buckwheat, or hot soaked and sifted rye porridge.

As much as I have wanted to consume breakfast cereals and granola again, I have not found one that I would consider healthy to consume on a regular basis. It's really a compromise food, no matter how many organic ingredients are on the label. The exception could be the 100 percent nut type of granolas that are made with soaked and dried nuts. But unfortunately for people with periodontal disease, a high nut intake is not recommended.

Soaking premade grain cereals like muesli overnight and consuming or cooking it with milk will make it a healthier option. The problem is that pre-flaked grains will likely oxidize, mold, or go rancid without refrigeration. There is also a problem of too much bran and germ when the entire grain is used. Hypothetically a good grain breakfast food might exist, yet I just could not recommend a store-bought product at the moment. Consider making a version yourself at home incorporating methods to remove the bran and break down the grain through soaking and souring.

Nuts and Nut Butters

As with grains, nuts are very high in plant toxins including phytic acid. For example, dogs are highly allergic to many types of nuts. The symptoms that dogs suffer from nut poisoning include muscle tremors, seizures, vomiting, diarrhea, drooling, and elevated heart rate. Nuts contain nourishing vitamins, but also potent plant toxins that could adversely affect the central nervous system. Some people with unhealthy teeth or gums rely too much on store-bought raw nut and seed butters as staples, such as too much raw tahini.

Nuts are powerful inhibitors of iron absorption,[28] and nuts contain about the same level of phytic acid as grains.[29] There are exceptions, for example even though fresh coconut has a moderate amount of phytic acid, fresh coconut has little or no impact on iron absorption. Sprouting nuts improves iron absorption, but only modestly. Vitamin C in the dose of at least twenty-five milligrams can prevent compounds in nuts from blocking iron absorption. Interestingly, the iron-blocking characteristics of nuts may have to do with how nut proteins are digested.[30] This may explain the indigenous cultures' propensity to mix nuts with animal proteins.

It seems almost universal that indigenous cultures either made oil with their nuts, or cooked their nuts in some way, such as adding them to meat soups and stews for their flavor and fat content. The general problem with nuts in the diet is that people often consume too many raw, and too much as a staple, rather than as a small part of a wholesome diet. An interesting note about macadamia nuts is that they are an aboriginal nut from Australia. Aboriginal peoples also had access to the highest vitamin C-rich fruit on the planet, the kakadu plum. Many types of macadamia nuts are known to be toxic and are not cultivated.

Since many people who are on grain-free diets consume coconut flour, I will mention that dried coconut flour has about the same amount of phytic acid, 1.17 percent,[31] as many grains and other nuts. Coconut does not impact iron absorption, which implies that it is much lower in plant toxins that are found in grains and beans. Traditional societies shred coconut and squeeze out the fat to produce the cherished coconut cream and coconut oil. Coconut flour is usually the by-product of coconut cream or coconut oil production, and coconut meal is usually used as animal feed. Even as an animal feed, its low protein digestibility causes pigs not to grow fully when it is used as a protein supplement.[32] It also contains twice the fiber of the bran of grains,[33] and high fiber diets, as previously discussed, tend to be irritating to the digestive tract and not conducive to health when used too much. Because of the phytic acid and fiber content of coconut flour, consuming it regularly may affect your calcium / phosphorous metabolism. I encourage moderation with coconut flour. If you do consume coconut flour, make sure to have plenty of phytic acid protecting factors like vitamin C.

Nut Suggestions

The problems with nuts for conditions of moderate to severe gum disease are multifold. First, nuts are very hard to chew and may irritate already sensitive gum tissues when eating them. Nuts are high in fat, and as discussed, a common problem for type-1 gum disease is a malabsorption of fat. Because nuts are both high in fat and high in potassium, they will likely aggravate imbalances in people with significant gum disease.

Nut Intake Suggestions

- ☐ If your gum disease is severe, consider avoiding nuts and seeds entirely.
- ☐ If your gum disease is less severe or you are improving, small amounts of nuts or

seeds used therapeutically would be okay. Just make nuts an occasional condiment in the diet and never a staple food.

Nut Intake to Maintain Health

- ☐ People who are healthy can consume nuts regularly with moderation.
    - ☐ Avoid commercially produced, non-organic nut butters.
    - ☐ Moderate the amount of nuts you eat; do not make them your staple food.
- ☐ Make sure to have plenty of food-based vitamin C, or calcium-rich foods with your nuts, such as roasted and skinless almonds with cheese, or nuts mixed with yogurt.

Additional Intermediate Guidelines

- ☐ Only consume nuts and nut butters that are soaked and dehydrated. (You can learn more about soaking nuts at curegumdisease.com/nuts.)

Advanced Nut Guidelines

- ☐ Roast nuts that have been soaked and use them for cooking, particularly with meat-based soups and stews.
    - ☐ Extract the oil from freshly roasted nuts.
- ☐ Or, avoid nuts entirely.

Avoid Sugar Like the Plague It Is!

Sugar and highly sweet foods are the worst possible foods to ingest if you have gum disease. The work of dentists Melvin Page and Weston Price show the disastrous effects of too much sugar in our diet. The more refined the sugar is, the more it is going to cause your blood sugar to fluctuate. The more extreme the fluctuation, the more disturbed your calcium and phosphorous metabolism. Fructose-containing sweeteners or sweeteners labeled as low glycemic may not raise your blood glucose level, but that does not make them safe because they raise your blood fructose levels. The end result is an even deeper disturbance in your calcium and phosphorous balance than what was caused by white sugar.[34, 35]

We already face the challenge of obtaining enough minerals in our diet. The more sweet foods we consume, the more we displace mineral-dense foods like pastured eggs, organ meats, seafood, and dairy foods.

As a summary, anything very sweet must be avoided if you want to get healthier. In particular, you must avoid and strictly limit any high intensity (very sweet) sweeteners like white sugar or high fructose corn syrup. This means anything that is or has a concentrated sweet flavor. While some sources of sweet are better than others, generally speaking, if it's too sweet, it is not good for you.

Common Sources of Sugar in Our Diet:

jam	"health food" bars	muffins
commercial honey	pastries	breakfast cereals
soda / soft drinks	ice cream	fruit juice
corn syrup	cookies	doughnuts
other syrups	toaster tarts	chocolate
sweetened drinks like iced tea	cake	sweetened coffee
candy		candy bars

I have received some complaints that the food protocols presented in *Cure Tooth Decay* are too strict or complicated to follow. My job is to share with you my best understanding of nature's principles for health so that you can activate your body's natural tooth and gum healing abilities. I also have to inform you that sugar will significantly cause and contribute to gum disease. How you take that information into your life is your choice. Knowing the connection between sugar and gum disease as discussed in chapter three should make it absolutely clear that the best results for healing for your mouth will be to incorporate a diet low in sweet foods.

While imported, exotic-sounding sweeteners may seem more appealing, at best they will affect the body the same as cane sugar, and at worst the effects will be far more detrimental. When large sums of money potentially can be made with every new sweetener on the market, companies selling sweeteners sometimes blur the lines of reality in order to sell more products and make more money. Just because the label presents a convincing marketing pitch does not mean you should be the next human guinea pig and test a new sweetener on yourself. Healthy sweeteners affect your blood sugar level. That is what sweet foods do. Sweeteners of industry, high in fructose, still disrupt the calcium and phosphorus metabolism. There is no free ride with sweeteners. You cannot have your sweets without a sacrifice to your body.

Evaporated Cane Juice and White Sugar – The empty calories from sugar provide energy, but do not provide nutrients to the body. White sugar will cause blood sugar fluctuations, which over time will result in mineral losses from your teeth and alveolar bone. Processed sugar consumption depletes chromium, zinc, magnesium, and manganese.[36] Health food product labels often list organic evaporated cane juice. Do not be fooled by this natural-sounding interpretation; this is still simply sugar. Sugar is recognized by the body, so it is far better than any of the artificial sugar replacements. If you are going to choose to buy a packaged food that is sweet, you want it to contain either sugar or fruit as a sweetener. **That being said, consuming sugar gives us calories that are not nutrient dense and will disrupt mineral metabolism.** The replacement of nutrient-dense foods with nutrient-poor sugar in our modern diet is in part what has contributed to tooth decay and gum disease with the rise of modern civilization.

High Fructose Corn Syrup (Corn Sugar) – This is by far the worst sweetener for our gums and overall health. Fructose in manmade products is not the same as fructose occurring naturally in fruit, and this often confuses people. A synthetic sugar and a natural sugar have been given the same name. Because high fructose corn syrup contains the synthetic form of fructose, it is toxic to the body. This explains why in study after study high fructose corn syrup is linked with serious diseases like pancreatic cancer, diabetes, and obesity.[37] My experience shows that consuming foods containing fructose is a recipe for glandular imbalances. High fructose corn syrup is part of the plague of the modern money-driven society. Manmade fructose is hiding in processed foods not just as corn syrup, but also under different aliases including the highly processed fructooligosaccharides (FOS) or inulin. These are both industrially produced sweeteners introduced into the market as low calorie sweeteners that are commonly mixed with high intensity sweeteners.[38] Sweetened drinks, soft drinks, and food bars are just a few of the foods commonly sweetened by fructose. The prevalence of the dangerous high fructose corn syrup in our foods is due to government subsidies to the corn industry, which make fructose cheaper to produce than natural sugar. This policy is not a good use of our tax dollars and in the long-run, it is making people very sick.

Xylitol – A research report in the *Journal of the American Dental Association* suggested that claims that xylitol stops cavities need further studies.[39] Xylitol's anti-cavity properties are purported to depend on the fact that bacteria cannot digest sugar alcohols and convert them into acids. Since it is clear that gum disease is not normally caused by bacteria, there is no reason to use this treatment for gum disease. Also avoid the other unnatural sounding sugar alcohol sweeteners such as sorbitol, mannitol, maltitol, and erythritol.

The Double Danger of Soft Drinks

Soft drinks contain high amounts of corn syrup and are highly acidic. They rob your body of calcium and magnesium once because of the corn syrup, and twice because of their acidity.

Agave Nectar – Agave nectar is a high-fructose-containing food masquerading as a health food. It contains as much or more fructose as high fructose corn syrup. Investigations have shown that agave nectar is not a raw or unrefined product despite marketing claims to the contrary.[40] Watch out, because agave nectar is hiding in many "health food" products such as "health food" bars. This makes many health food bars mere candy bars made with industrially produced sweeteners. Consumers are largely in the dark when left to choose between products marketed as "health" foods, and what is truly healthy to eat—pure and unrefined foods.

Glycerin – Once a by-product of candle making, this sweetener now comes from a variety of sources including biodiesel manufacturing.[41] Although glycerin has many uses, it is a sweetener that I avoid and do not recommend for regular consumption.

Malted Grain Sweeteners – Watch out for malted grain sweeteners like malted barley and corn. People consuming these sweeteners have reported tooth decay, which means they are losing minerals when consuming these sweeteners. The detrimental mineral imbalances may likely be caused by the type of the sugars in the grain or the plant toxins from the grain.[42]

Brown Rice Syrup – The human body can recognize the sugar in brown rice syrup. However, I am very concerned about the presence of grain anti-nutrients, and the enzyme methodology of processing and creating the syrup. Brown rice syrup is similar to malted barley syrup, which people's reports indicate can significantly promote cavities and therefore it should be avoided.[43]

Molasses – This by-product of beet or cane sugar production probably is about as safe as cane sugar in relation to gum disease. It may be acceptable for specific therapeutic use, but not for regular use.

Sugar Isolates – Maltodextrin, sucrose, dextrose, and so forth are isolates of naturally occurring sugars and are commonly found in processed foods. At best, their effects disrupt mineral levels as much as regular sugar; at worst, they are far worse.[44]

Fake Sweeteners – These are sucralose, aspartame, and saccharine. A wide body of evidence and concern exists regarding the hazards of artificial sweeteners.

For further information about toxic sugars, visit **sugarshockblog.com.**

The longer your blood sugar is out of control, the longer and more significantly the calcium and phosphorus ratios are altered, and the greater the likelihood of gum recession and inflammation. Regardless of whether the sugar is white sugar or sugar from fruit consumption, it still affects your blood sugar level. If sweet foods, or sweeteners, natural or processed, are consumed several times per day, then the alteration in blood sugar will be prolonged and consistent. Over time, this will lead to a consistent alteration of blood calcium and phosphorous levels and likely cause gum disease.

Below is a summary of sweeteners to avoid due to their ability to cause alternations in blood sugar or blood chemistry.[45] Even if a sweetener is not listed here, do not eat it if you do not know exactly what it is.

white sugar
cane sugar
evaporated cane juice
xylitol
agave nectar
jams
dried fruit
candy bars
health food bars
yacon syrup
lo han
palm sugar
coconut sugar
stevia extract
glycerin
fructose
high fructose corn syrup
inulin
fructooligosaccharides (FOS)
erythritol
malted barley
grain sweeteners
maltodextrin
sucrose
dextrose
sucralose
aspartame
saccharine
brown rice syrup

Fruit and Your Health

Fruit, particularly berries, can add to your health. But too much fruit means too much sugar, and that can contribute to gum recession by causing excess blood sugar fluctuations. Most of the fruit on store shelves today is hybridized. For example, an ancient apple was a small, not very sweet fruit, which probably needed to be cooked to be edible. But many decades of cultivation, selection, and hybridization have created large juicy apples with high sugar content. While fruit is natural, the high sugar content of most modern fruits means that many people cannot eat as much fruit as they want and remain healthy. Fruit is not a bad food choice, but many people eat too much. Many people have mistakenly made fruit a staple item of their diets, rather than seeing it as a snack, side dish, or occasional treat.

Fruit is best eaten with fat. Fruit and cream go well together, such as peaches or strawberries with cream. Some fruit goes well with cheese, such as apples or pears. Some people consume excess amounts of very sweet fruits. The sugar in these fruits helps calm hunger by providing rapid energy. But fruit does not give the body sufficient nutrient building blocks like protein. Sweet fruits commonly consumed include oranges, peaches, grapes, and tropical fruits such as pineapple and bananas. I highly recommend limiting these very sweet fruits when you are trying to halt gum recession. Gum disease is directly correlated with blood sugar imbalances, and eating excessive natural sweets will not allow your system to correct itself. Once gum disease is a distant memory, you can safely eat more sweet fruits. For some people, cooking all of their fruit before eating it is helpful as it transforms the sugars and can increase digestibility. Fruits are also generally picked before they are ripe, which can increase salicylate content, which some people are sensitive to.

Basic fruit recommendations: Avoid or greatly limit highly sweet fruits like dates, peaches, pineapples, dried fruit, blueberries, and bananas until your gum recession has completely healed.

Intermediate fruit recommendations: Only enjoy fruit once a day around the middle of the day such as after lunch. Fruit and sweeteners eaten later in the day can make it difficult to get restful sleep, or make it harder to fall asleep. And sound sleep is important for healing the body. The fruit you do eat should not be too sweet. Examples of less sweet fruits are less sweet berries, such as raspberries, and green apples.

Advanced fruit recommendations: If you have severe periodontal disease, consider avoiding all sweets and fruits completely and see how you feel.

Safer Sweeteners in Moderation

Use these following sweeteners in moderation when you do not have active periodontal disease. With active periodontal disease and symptoms like loose teeth, bleeding gums, and infectious gum pockets, make every effort to temporarily avoid all added sweets. In my family, we typically do not eat anything sweet besides a little bit of fruit once or twice a day, such as an apple with some cheese. A few times per week we use small amounts of unheated honey, or grade B (very dark/strong taste) organic maple syrup. Two to four times per month we make something with a little more sweetness as a special treat.

Unheated honey – Choose honey that states it is unheated, or never heated, on the label. Bees work very hard to keep their hive at around ninety-three degrees Fahrenheit. If the hive gets too hot, the bees abandon the hive. Ideally, honey should be harvested at or below ninety-three degrees. Honey that is labeled as "raw," but does not state unheated or never heated, may have been heated to a much higher temperatures than ninety-three degrees, and many of the benefits of the honey may be lost. For this reason, honey is not good for cooking. Despite the claims of some manufacturers of honey, honey does not prevent tooth decay or gum disease. It is however an excellent sweetener if it is the genuine article. A common practice for beekeepers is to feed the bees a sugar supplement so they produce more honey. Make sure the honey you buy is made in the U.S. and not from supplemented bees. Real honey will become cloudy or crystallize after a few days or weeks from bottling or the bottle being opened.[46]

Maple Syrup – Grade B (very dark/strong taste) organic maple syrup will have your body saying "yes." Beware, though, because many maple syrups—even some labeled organic—contain formaldehyde residue from the illegal practice of using formaldehyde pellets to keep tap holes open in trees. I have felt sick from a generic brand of organic maple syrup, so I now choose smaller independent brands that are more likely to be using the best practices. Even better than maple syrup is maple sugar, which is a traditional sweetener, used by native peoples in the Northeast. Note: Grade A and Grade B maple syrups are extremely similar and are processed in the same way, the difference is the color.[47] Grade B (very dark/strong taste) feels like it absorbs a little slower than Grade A, so I prefer Grade B.

Real Cane Sugar – In ancient Ayurveda, real sugar such as jaggery is considered a medicine.[48] But most of the sugar available in grocery stores today is far from medicinal. Most varieties are excessively processed. Safer forms of sugar are pure cane juice, if you have access to fresh sugar cane; Heavenly Organics ™ Sugar; or Rapunzel's Rapadura sugar. As far as I know, other sugars labeled raw, organic, or anything else are likely to be significantly processed, with the minerals removed. Both cane sugar and maple syrup can be safely used in cooking.

Stevia (Use extreme caution) – Stevia is a very sweet herb. You must be extremely careful with its use because it may have other medicinal properties besides its use as a sweetener. Many sweeteners are made from extracting components of the stevia leaf; extracts of stevia will likely cause calcium / phosphorous imbalances. The only stevia that is safe to use is the ground dried herb that is fresh stevia that is simply dried and powdered. **I do not recommend stevia at this time for people with severe gum disease.[49]**

Avoid Toxic Fat

When modern industry and commerce blighted the diets of native peoples across the globe, most people reduced their consumption of natural animal fats in favor of industrially processed vegetable oils. Since animal fats are a key source of fat-soluble vitamins, this change resulted in a loss of the crucial fat-soluble vitamins in the diet. Unfortunately, most restaurants today also use cheap, refined vegetable oils for cooking. When I consume these oils I do not feel well and suffer cold and flu-like symptoms of congestion.

Trans Fats - *Trans* fats are produced by adding hydrogen to vegetable oil through a process called hydrogenation. Margarine is an example of a trans fat, although not all margarines today contain trans fats. Factory made trans fats are toxic to the body.[50] Trans fats have replaced saturated real fats like organic butter, tallow, and lard.[51]

Canola Oil – Canola is not the name of a plant, but rather a shortened term for "Canada oil." The FDA prohibits the use of canola oil in baby formulas because it retards growth.[52] The trans fat content of canola oil is listed at 0.2 percent, yet independent research has found trans levels as high as 4.6 percent in commercial liquid oil.[53] Canola oil is extracted by a combination of high temperature mechanical pressing and solvent extraction. My experience in consuming canola oil is that it makes me feel congested and I start coughing. Because it is cheap and believed to be healthy due to its monounsaturated lipid content, canola oil is what many restaurants and health food stores use for cooking and frying foods. If they only knew that this toxic oil was harming their customers they might stop using it. These establishments tout the health benefits of canola oil, yet may lose out on return business by not using tastier animal fats.

Safflower, soy, and corn oils are all on the list of oils to avoid. Because of their delicate structure, these vegetable oils are especially dangerous after being heated in the process of cooking or frying.[54] A more recent study linked a high safflower oil diet to obesity and diabetes.[55]

Avoid other low quality vegetable oils including soybean and hydrogenated cottonseed oil, and any food not fried in a natural fat. Watch out for store-bought potato chips, which are usually fried in oils that are not suitable for health.

Most restaurants use discount vegetable oils. While many choose these oils because they are cheap, they are definitely not healthy. Even if a restaurant says they use olive oil or duck fat, you have to ask them if it is 100 percent. Too often healthy oils are purposely diluted with cheaper oils to lower restaurant costs. Unfortunately store-bought low cost olive oil, even labeled as pure, is often adulterated with other oils.[56]

Healthy Fats

Healthy fats support balanced hormonal function and they are also a great source of energy. They come from organic plant sources and include avocado, palm, coconut, and olive oil. Healthy animal fats come from free-range animals consuming their natural diet and include butter, lard, tallow, and schmaltz (rendered chicken, goose, or duck fat).

Nut and Seed Oils

Nut and seed oils have been a part of the human diet for a very long time. Walnut oil is popular in France and Italy as a salad dressing. For the nut oils to be healthy, many of them require careful processing, or fresh pressing. Limit or avoid nut and seed oils (such as expeller pressed) as best you can unless they are from small artisan producers.

Avoid Low Quality Proteins and Vegetables

Native peoples generally consumed all parts of the animals they hunted or fished, including, and often preferentially, the organs such as liver, kidney, brain, and heart. Plant foods were eaten in prime condition either freshly prepared, fermented to enhance nutrient content, or preserved using time-tested methods of drying and fermenting. By contrast, foods prominent in the modern industrial diet are devitalized by industrial processing. Tinned meats and vegetables undergo high heat and pressure in the canning process, which damages protein quality and also destroys many vitamins and all enzymes naturally present in the fresh or fermented versions.

Low Quality Proteins

Factory-farmed meats and eggs promote a profit-driven system of disease. The cesspools from these factory farms pollute the air and the environment including water supplies. Factory-farmed animals are concentrated in restricted indoor housing and barely allowed to move, are loaded with drugs and chemicals to keep them alive, and are not fed their natural diet. It is unwise to eat the unhealthy meat from these animals. Choose fresh grass-fed or organic meats whenever possible. Choose wild fish whenever possible, as farm-raised fish are not fed their natural diet. Mollusks like oysters can be wild farmed, and those are safe to eat so long as the water is clean.

Conventional packaged lunch meats contain many harmful food additives. My experience is that store-bought preserved meats such as salami, bacon, and hot dogs are not health promoting. Use cured and prepared meat products with care. Even if they are labeled as organic, they may be hard for the body to digest. Opt instead for freshly made sausages and artisan-produced aged meat products.

Protein Powders

There are three types of commonly used protein powders, and care needs to be taken with all of them. Soy protein contains toxic substances and blocks iron absorption even when all of the phytic acid has been removed.[57] Hemp protein powder is made from the waste products left over from the manufacture of hemp oil from hemp seeds. It is unclear if hemp seeds have anti-nutrients or not; if you have gum disease, I would use this with caution. Avoid protein powders from phytate-rich grains like brown rice. Many low quality protein powders are loaded with sweeteners of various sorts and the sugar sweetened powder will cause deleterious blood sugar fluctuations.

Protein is best obtained from pasture-fed animal foods and eggs, as well as wild seafood and insects. Many people use protein powder to significantly increase their protein intake beyond what they can obtain from a healthy diet. This excessive protein intake could be imbalancing to the body. However, if for a specific reason you need a protein powder, look for a low temperature dried, unflavored, grass-fed whey without any additives. But be cautious, as many protein powders on the market are overly processed, unhealthy / toxic, and use inferior ingredients. Further research is required at this time to give definitive answers about this, so I am not encouraging its use, but I understand that it can be useful for specific reasons.

Soy Products Can Be Toxic

A friend of mine thought eating large amounts of tofu was a good idea. In a short time, her hair began falling out and her skin turned pale. Soy contains plant hormones that need to be disabled through a careful fermentation process, which tofu does not undergo. High levels of phytic acid in soy reduce the assimilation of calcium, magnesium, copper, iron, and zinc. Phytic acid in soy is not neutralized by ordinary preparation methods such as soaking, sprouting, and long, slow cooking. High phytate diets have caused growth problems in children.[58] Not all soy foods are troublesome, however. Unpasteurized fermented soy sauce (shoyu), traditionally made miso paste, organic tempeh (use with moderation), and natto are all long-fermented soy dishes and are safe to consume for most people in moderation.

Take Care with Substitute Milks

Soy milk contains enzyme inhibitors and high levels of plant estrogens. Avoid store-bought soy milk.

Store-bought **rice milk** and nut milks may contain large amounts of grain and nut anti-nutrients like phytic acid or oxalates. Although it may not say it on the label, rice bran may be the main ingredient of some rice milks. The more serious issue with these processed "milks" is their high levels of sugar.

Nut and seed milks may also contain high concentrations of plant toxins so I do not recommend you buy them from the store. Nuts are highly prized by native groups for their oils, and nut milk can be made at home. Yet homemade milks may still contain anti-nutrients or plant toxins if they are not thoroughly cooked. Use nut milk with care.

Suggestion: If you are a rice milk or nut milk lover, make it at home yourself. In general consider using recipes that use cooked ingredients, or involve heating or fermentation. Do not settle for cheap imitations.

Give up the Coffee Habit

Coffee stimulates our glands to secrete hormones that cause our livers to release stored sugar and energy. The frequent use of coffee wears out the pancreas and its blood sugar balancing functions. Usually people drink coffee as a means to lift their depleted energy without consuming food.[59] This process wears on the nutrient stores in your body, and likely contributes to calcium loss.[60] Coffee may also acidify your body chemistry, which is counterproductive in the case of gum disease, when a more alkaline status is desired. Coffee can destroy vitamin C in the body as well as deplete the body of vitamin B12.[61] Historically coffee enemas have been an excellent way to detoxify the liver, so if you are addicted to coffee, perhaps you are "drinking" it in the wrong way.

Tea

Caffeinated tea affects the body in ways similar to coffee, just not quite as harsh.[62] Limit or avoid caffeinated teas, which are often found contaminated with pesticides. Nowadays there are many herbal blends that can replace caffeinated teas. Most non-caffeinated herbal teas will be beneficial to your health provided their purpose is to nourish and not to stimulate. Two examples of nourishing herbal teas would be nettle tea and red raspberry leaf tea.

Smoking

Cigar, pipe, and cigarette smoking is a significant risk factor for periodontal disease and tooth loss.[63] If you smoke and suffer periodontal disease you will need to quit in order to heal.

Beer and Wine

Sorry to report some bad news to the home brewers and beer aficionados out there. The excessive use of alcohol is as disastrous as white sugar and white flour to your body chemistry. Beer consumption increases the acidity of the body, increases blood levels of phosphorous, and promotes the excretion of calcium. Healthy individuals can enjoy beer and wine in moderation. But if you are suffering from gum disorders, it is best to avoid alcohol, as it is an enemy of calcium metabolism and utilization.[64] The desire for alcohol could be caused by a glandular imbalance,[65] a lack of fermented foods, or a deficiency in calories or nutrients.

Table Salt

Pure white table salt is sodium chloride extracted from its associated minerals. It has anti-caking ingredients and iodine added. As long as you eat some kelp powder you will get plenty of iodine. Table salt is overly refined and seems toxic to most people.[66] A suitable alternative is unrefined sea salt.

High Fat and High Potassium Foods

High fat and high potassium foods are associated with gum disease. Some foods that are high in both fat and potassium are nuts, doughnuts, and chocolate.[67] Dr. Hawkins warned against many high potassium foods in relation to gum disease including: bananas, chocolate, honey, fruit juice, dried fruits, nuts, molasses, olives, potatoes, wheat bran, and soft drinks.

Fruit Juice and Sweetened Beverages

Because gum disease is intimately tied with high blood sugar, fruit juice should be avoided. Fruit juice tends to lower muscle tone, reduce the calcium level of the body, decrease the hydrochloric acid of the stomach, and cause acidosis of the body.[68]

Health food stores sell many sweetened and protein-fortified vegetable and fruit juices. The pasteurization process damages important nutrients and cell structures and removes a significant amount of healing ability that these juices might otherwise provide. Store-bought juices are full of sugar, whether added or naturally occurring, and, sorry to say, it is just too much for those susceptible to gum disease. Sweet drinks loaded with sugar provide empty calories. Here and there a naturally fermented drink that is a little bit sweet like real kombucha will not do you much harm if you do not have gum recession. Watch out in particular for sports drinks and sweetened teas. Replace these with unsweetened herbal teas, raw milk, whey, or kefir.

Birth Control Pills and Gingival Bleeding

Oral contraceptives have long been considered a risk factor for gingival bleeding, and users of birth control pills have poorer oral health than women who do not use them.[69] Fertility awareness method (FAM) or natural family planning (NFP) are alternatives that don't require synthetic hormones, but they do require significant attention to details because mistakes can often result in pregnancy. Birth control pills often cause copper toxicity. Eating plenty of zinc-rich food like oysters will help balance out the imbalances caused by birth control pills.

MSG and Hormonal Balance

Consuming monosodium glutamate (MSG) may alter your endocrine gland balance and contribute to gum disease. Most store-bought soups, sauces, and broth mixes contain MSG, either as an added ingredient or a residue of hydrolyzation and other industrial food processing methods. MSG shows up secretly in product labels under different names. Avoid products containing the following ingredients: hydrolyzed vegetable protein (HVP), textured protein, yeast extract, autolyzed plant protein, and anything with the word glutamate or glutamic acid.

Fluoride Causes Gum Recession

Fluoride toothpaste carries a warning notice against swallowing the product because fluoride is poisonous. The same fluoride that is in toothpaste is used as a rat poison. Fluoride is a chemical poison placed in about 66 percent of the U.S. water supplies with the claim that it prevents dental cavities. The World Health Organization has published a study showing that there is no decrease in cavity levels in countries that fluoridate their water supplies compared with those that do not.[70]

The highest rates of tooth loss from periodontal disease in people over the age of sixty occur in the regions with the highest rates of water fluoridation. Increased fluoride exposure results in an increase in periodontal disease and dental fluorosis.71 To find out if your water is fluoridated, call your water department. If you do live in a fluoridated area, consider getting a bottled water delivery service or a multi-stage fluoride filter to purify your water. To learn more about the dangers of fluoride and what you can do about it, visit fluoridealert.org.

Prescription Drugs and Gum Disease

Certain types of pharmaceutical drugs are recognized in the periodontal literature as causing or contributing to gum disease. These include calcium channel blockers as well as immunomodulatory drugs, anticonvulsants, and many other drugs such as those that result in dry mouth or reduce saliva flow.[72] Any drug that affects the thyroid gland can also affect the calcium / phosphorous metabolism and thus lead to gum recession. In addition to the types of drugs mentioned, any habitually used prescription drug many contribute to glandular imbalances leading to periodontal disease. If you change your diet and find you are not improving, then prescription drugs may be the cause. If this is the case, work closely with your doctor to both lower your prescription and find an effective alternative non-pharmaceutical treatment.

Electromagnetic Smog Contributes to Neuroendocrine Stress

In chapter three I discussed the work of Dr. Page and how stress can disturb the balance of our neuroendocrine system in states of disease. Our body runs on electrical currents of energy. Cells vibrate and talk to one another via very subtle electrical pulses. An EKG is an example of monitoring the electrical pulse of the heart. Electromagnetic fields (EMFs) produced by modern technologies create frequencies and patterns that affect our body in unnatural ways. Think of EMFs like X-rays. We cannot feel an X-ray, but we know that the radiation is harmful and that it should be limited and avoided if possible.

EMFs are emitted not only from cell phones, but also from the walls of our houses as the electrical systems in our homes run at high frequency oscillations. Dangers of EMFs have been hidden from the U.S. population because the electronics industry sets their own standards for EMF safety. Pollution from cell phones, computer devices, Wi-Fi, and wireless technologies all add significantly to our levels of environmental stress. If you are new to the concept of electromagnetic pollution, then it might seem peculiar that something that cannot be felt, and that is utterly ubiquitous, would have any negative effects. By contrast, the governments of Germany and Switzerland advise their public schools not to use Wi-Fi[73] because electromagnetic fields have been shown to produce negative health effects, especially for children.

Here are some simple steps to reduce EMFs:

- Turn off the house power in your bedroom at night.
- Turn off the Wi-Fi in your house when you are not using it and when you sleep. Alternatively, switch to wired Internet.
- Reduce wireless radiation by turning your phone off, keeping it away from your body, using an earpiece, not holding the phone near your head, and buying a Pong or equivalent radiation cell phone protector which can be found through this link: curegumdisease.com/emf.
- Purchase a few Graham-Stetzer Filters to reduce whole house EMF fields, learn more at: curegumdisease.com/emf.

An important consideration is that EMF fields and metal poisoning in the body can react together. So if you suffer mercury or heavy metals toxicity, the effects of EMFs can be far greater than for those without such burdens. For more information about the severe and serious dangers of EMFs, visit curegumdisease.com/emf.

Mercury Fillings Are a Significant Risk Factor in Gum Disease

Mercury is a highly toxic substance put in people's mouths. The silver colored amalgam fillings are approximately 50 percent mercury.

Mercury poisoning has been linked to gum disease as early as 1917.[74] Historically mercury has been used as a medicine, and a known side effect of mercury poisoning was gum disease, resulting in loose teeth and significant infection.[75] A large and recent German study found a significant relationship between the number of amalgam fillings and gum disease.[76] In another study of people poisoned by mercury fillings, about half of them had the symptom is bleeding gums. In the months and years following amalgam removal, half of the patients with bleeding gums had the symptoms completely eliminated.[77]

Scientific literature has shown mercury fillings can cause:

- Gum tissue inflammation
- Bleeding gums

- ☐ Metal taste in mouth
- ☐ Chronic inflammation
- ☐ Lichen planus (itchy rash that can be in or around the mouth)

Mercury fillings give off toxic mercury vapor and can cause amalgam tattoos, which are grey or black spots on our gums where mercury has leached into the tissue.

Mercury fillings can amplify electrical currents in the body to levels as high as one thousand times stronger than those optimal for the central nervous system. This can contribute to parasympathetic suppression or sympathetic dominance.[78] Oral galvanism is a condition in which dissimilar metals in the mouth (such as gold and mercury) create electrical currents as well as higher levels of mercury vapor.[79] Having two different metals in the mouth occurs when metal crowns cover a mercury filling, or with titanium implants as the implant and crown on the implant can be made of different materials. As if mercury was not toxic enough to the body, galvanic currents produced by dissimilar metals make matters worse. Dissimilar metals can cause health symptoms that doctors cannot resolve and their cause is often missed. The symptoms include brain fog, confusion, migraine headache, dizziness, and digestive problems.[80] Indeed a large U.S. Centers for Disease Control study found that those with mercury fillings had more chronic health conditions.[81]

Mercury in the teeth can travel and leach directly into the brain and central nervous system. Direct routes from the teeth and gums to the brain suggest mercury can be a significant cause or factor in Alzheimer's disease.[82] Dentist Mark Breiner, author of *Whole Body Dentistry,* wrote that, "You would be amazed at how many patients' gums stopped bleeding after the patients have their mercury fillings removed."[83]

If you have or have had mercury fillings, then it is reasonable to assume that you have some heavy metal poisoning. If you eat reasonably well but still have digestive problems, it is possible that heavy metals are the cause.[84]

Clearly mercury is highly toxic to the body and is highly correlated with gum disease along with digestive problems. Mercury poisoning significantly inhibits many of the body's normal functions and places a significant strain on the body, resulting in bleeding gums and other symptoms that would be labeled as gum disease. Indeed, many cases of gum disease are symptoms of mercury poisoning.

Vaccines and Calcium Metabolism

Toxic metals such as mercury, aluminum, cadmium, arsenic, lead, and nickel can interfere with calcium and phosphorus entering the cells.[85] So to stay healthy, it is important to avoid these toxic metals. And if your health is out of balance, it is possible that besides mercury poisoning, that you may have metal poisoning from other sources, including a source perhaps you did not expect, vaccines. Strangely, toxic metals are added to vaccines to trap the vaccine substances (virus, etc.) in the body, otherwise they are flushed out. Getting vaccines such as the annual flu vaccine puts us at risk for heavy metal poisoning. The flu vaccine is loaded with mercury, and is therefore extremely poisonous.[86] Vaccines also contain many neurological poisons. Vaccine ingredients include ethylene glycol (antifreeze), formaldehyde, aluminum, thimerosal (mercury), neomycin (antibiotic), streptomycin (antibacterial), squalene (fish or plant oil), MSG, and phenol (a caustic, poisonous acidic compound present in coal tar and wood tar).[87] The question for you to consider is if these ingredients are unfit to eat, then what happens when they are directly injected into our bloodstream? There are many books that educate about the dangers of vaccines. I personally do not take them or recommend them. The last vaccine I got twenty years ago, when I did not know better, was a tetanus vaccine loaded with mercury that made me quite ill. Since toxic metals contribute to gum disease, to help stop gum disease you need to avoid more sources of toxic metals. I have a web resource to direct you to accurate and detailed sources where you can learn about vaccine toxins and how to avoid them at: curegumdisease.com/vaccines.

Chapter Six Summary

I recommend that regarding lifestyle you:

- ☐ Quit smoking, if you smoke.
- ☐ Reduce EMFs, whenever possible.
- ☐ Avoid oral contraceptives.
- ☐ Avoid fluoride in our water and toothpaste.
- ☐ Consider the impact of mercury in your mouth.
- ☐ Avoid vaccines that contain toxic metals as well as other neurological poisons.

I recommend that regarding nutrition you:

- ☐ Avoid MSG, which may be listed as: hydrolyzed vegetable protein (HVP), textured protein, yeast extract, autolyzed plant protein, and anything with the word glutamate or glutamic acid.
- ☐ Avoid bleached white flour products or and/or non-organic grains.
- ☐ Avoid commercially made whole grain products.
- ☐ Avoid sprouted grain breads.
- ☐ Avoid most gluten-free grain products.
- ☐ Avoid health food bars.
- ☐ Avoid breakfast cereals and store-bought granola, organic or otherwise.
- ☐ Avoid a high and seed nut intake. Only consume nuts that have been soaked and dehydrated first. If gum disease is severe, avoid nuts and seeds altogether.
- ☐ Avoid trans fat and vegetable oils such as canola, safflower, soy, and corn. In their place, consume avocado, palm, coconut, and olive oil, as well as butter, lard, tallow, and schmaltz (rendered chicken, goose, or duck fat) from animals on pasture. Avoid conventional packaged lunch meats.
- ☐ Avoid protein powders.
- ☐ Avoid all soy products with the exception unpasteurized fermented soy sauce (shoyu), traditionally made miso paste, organic tempeh, and natto in moderation.
- ☐ Avoid milk substitutes.
- ☐ Avoid coffee and caffeinated tea.
- ☐ Avoid fruit juice.
- ☐ Avoid table salt. Consume unrefined sea salt instead.
- ☐ Avoid sugar in any form.
- ☐ Limit unheated honey, maple syrup, real cane sugar. Use extreme caution with stevia.
- ☐ Limit fruit consumption, and eat it with fat, such as an apple with cheese.
- ☐ Limit popcorn.
- ☐ Limit coconut flour, and have it with plenty of vitamin C in your diet.
- ☐ Limit or avoid nut and seed oils (such as expeller pressed) as best you can unless they are from small artisan producers.
- ☐ Limit alcohol such as beer and wine.

- ☐ Choose fresh grass-fed or organic meats whenever possible. Choose wild fish whenever possible as farm-raised fish are not fed their natural diet. Mollusks like oysters can be wild farmed, and those are safe to eat so long as the water is clean.

Keep in mind:

1. One recipe for creating gum disease is a diet high in meat and grains and low in calcium from dairy products. A diet that heavily favors meat and grains and is also low in calcium is disproportionately high in phosphorus and can contribute to a calcium/phosphorus imbalance in the body that may lead to gum disease.
2. Grains need to be properly prepared via sourdough techniques or soaking to be a nourishing food. Ideally, when applicable, they would be freshly ground and sifted to remove the bran and germ before being used.
3. Gluten-free grains can still contain calcium-leaching anti-nutrients like phytic acid, in addition gluten-free products typically contain cheap oils, fillers, soy, and other unsavory ingredients that we recommend you avoid.
4. Adults with gum problems would do well to avoid grains for two to three weeks to let their bodies recover and find balance. When you consume grains, nuts, seeds, or beans regularly, make sure to include adequate calcium, vitamin C, and vitamin D in your diet.
5. Beans can be delicious foods, but they can also contain many plant toxins. Beans are high in phytic acid and lectins. Soaking beans overnight in a slightly alkaline solution (using a pinch of baking soda for example) and then cooking them eliminates a good portion of phytic acid in smaller beans like lentils. Lentils without the bran are probably the safest beans to eat. Take the same food combining precautions with beans as you would with grains. Eat beans with cheese or yogurt, vitamin D-containing-foods, and vitamin C-rich vegetables. Cooking beans with kombu (sea kelp) makes the beans more digestible.
6. Regarding sweets, keep in mind that gum disease is directly correlated with blood sugar imbalances and eating excessive natural sweets, in the form of fruit and honey for example, will not allow your system to correct itself.
7. Dr. Hawkins warned against many high potassium foods in relation to gum disease including: bananas, chocolate, honey, fruit juice, dried fruits, nuts, molasses, olives, potatoes, wheat bran, and soft drinks.
8. Gum disease is the result of nutrient deficiencies.

7 Good Digestion is Necessary for Healthy Gums

Nutritional deficiencies have at least three causes:

1. The right foods are not being consumed and so there is a shortfall of the needed vitamins and minerals.
2. Toxic foods, industrial foods, and environmental toxins like heavy metals or lifestyle stresses burden the body and deplete the minerals that we already have.
3. The vitamins and minerals consumed are not being absorbed and properly utilized.

In addition to making the right food choices, we need to be able to digest, assimilate, and utilize the nutrients in the foods that we eat. If you cannot digest or assimilate your food well, your healing results may be less than optimal.

The Cause of Disease Including Gum Disease

Many people with gum disease do not digest food well. The symptoms of poor digestion include gas, constipation, diarrhea, burping, burning sensations, vomiting, indigestion, bloating, and pain after eating.[1] The science of Ayurveda developed by the physicians and seers of ancient India states that indigestion and food malabsorption are the primary causes of all disease, which includes gum disease. According to Ayurveda, the four main factors of that cause disease are:

1. **Incomplete digestion** (known as ama) occurs when food is not broken down properly and results in partially digested material. Ayurvedic medicine practitioners think the root cause of all disease is incompletely digested food (ama) that is not eliminated by the body. Partially digested food can make us feel heavy and sluggish after eating.
2. **Putrefaction** (known as amavisha; visha means poison) occurs when incompletely digested food in the body is not excreted. It becomes putrefied and rancid like rotting vegetables and turns very acidic in the body. This toxic undigested

food clogs the body and results in systemic stiffness and inflammation. This is likely the primary cause of an acid pH in the mouth and the high levels of inflammation associated with gum disease.

3. **Poisoning** (known as garavisha) happens when a poisonous substance coming from sources outside of the body damages the body tissues. Examples of noxious substances in the environment include poisonous mushrooms, chemicals, pesticides, and food additives, as well as mercury, lead, and other toxic metals.
4. **Electromagnetic Field Poison** (known as Indravajravijanyavisha) is a poison caused by exposure to electrical fields, or EMFs.[2] Ayurveda identified this as a source of disease more than a thousand years ago.

Because toxic substances and electrical fields have the potential to significantly affect our health and inhibit healing, discussions of mercury poisoning and EMFs have been included in this book because they can both affect your overall health as well as your ability to digest and metabolize food.

Good Digestion Is Essential to Gum Health

If you eat nourishing food as described in this book but still suffer from gum disease, you likely also suffer from at least one of the following: acid reflux, gall bladder problems, kidney disease, diabetes, or another health challenge that contributes to digestive interference.[3] Toxins from undigested foods not only cause inflammation in the body, but also interfere with the absorption and utilization of minerals from food and supplements.

Let's briefly examine digestion to help clarify what is happening. The digestive process is the breakdown of food into vitamins, energy, and nutrition for our body to function. It begins when we start to think about what food we want to eat, or what we are about to eat. When food is taken in the mouth, salivary enzymes and chewing begin the breakdown process. The food is then propelled down the throat to the stomach, which is a highly acidic environment that has an acid pH of 1.5–3.5. Along with the highly acidic stomach acid, the stomach mechanically churns the food that was swallowed. After digesting in the stomach, the food passes through the pyloric valve to the first part of the small intestine, the duodenum.

The liver creates a more alkaline digestive substance, bile, which has a greenish yellow color and is stored in the gall bladder and helps specifically with fat digestion along with overall digestion. During digestion, the acidic chime, the mass produced by the stomach, is mixed with both bile, from the liver, and enzymes, from the pancreas, to break down fats, proteins, and carbohydrates. It is the healthy combi-

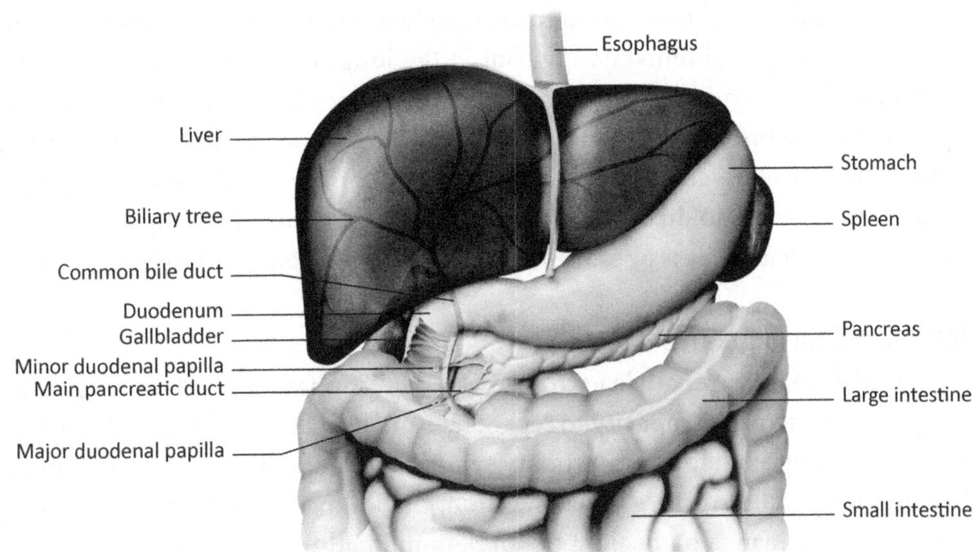

nation of these substances that breaks food down enough for it to be absorbed in the small intestine. As food in our body remains warm, it eventually ferments in the large intestine, where bacteria further break down the food and create vitamins. And after a while, out it comes.

Digestive Problems Underlie Many Dietary Habits and Paradigms

People who digest protein poorly tend to gravitate toward vegetarian or vegan diets because they have noticed, subconsciously or consciously, that too much animal protein makes them feel ill. Similarly, people gravitate to low-carbohydrate (carb) diets when they digest carbohydrates poorly. When fat digestion is a problem, high-carb, low fat diets may seem like a panacea. In each case, people who restrict major food categories in their diets have not likely found a "perfect diet," but rather, have eliminated a source of toxic undigested food from their body.

This is why some people report amazing health benefits from fasting on vegetable juices and raw green vegetable smoothies, while others thrive from avoiding starchy carbohydrates and eating bacon, red meat, butter, and cream. While a specialized diet based on food avoidance may help in the shorter term, in the long run, abstaining or restricting too much of any food category leads to disease, weakness, and poor health. That is why many long-time vegetarians or vegans return to eating meat. And this is also why some people who follow extreme carbohydrate restriction feel happier when they eventually return to eating carbohydrate foods.

To summarize, a short term (approximately one to four weeks) specialized diet may be cleansing and rejuvenating. But in the long run, dietary dogmas tend to become inflexible and overly limit their dietary choices, and as a result, people end up depriving themselves. If over a sustained period of time the diet you are eating is not making you feel well, then a careful assessment of your food choices and appropriate adjustments should be made, rather than assume you are doing it wrong and to keep trying harder. It is possible that the paradigm itself is not right for you.

Increase Your Digestive Potency

Increased digestive strength leads to decreased inflammation, greater energy, and a body with an increased capacity to regenerate and heal. An acidic pH in the mouth caused by undigested food is a primary symptom of gum disease and tooth decay. Because it is vital to restore your digestion, the following suggestions may help. For detailed guidance on healing the organs and pathways of digestion, consider working closely with an alternative medicine physician or other licensed holistic health care practitioner such as a naturopath, acupuncturist, chiropractor, Ayurvedic practitioner, and so forth. It is up to you to find someone whom you trust to provide the guidance and support you need.

Simple Suggestions for Better Digestion

Organic Apple Cider Vinegar. Take approximately half a teaspoon or more in a half cup of warm water twice per day, ideally after waking and before bed. Some people benefit from as much as three tablespoons of apple cider vinegar diluted in water per day. This helps promote healthy stomach acidity. (Using a straw may help conserve tooth enamel for sensitive people.)

The Spice of Life. For thousands of years, spices have been treasured as digestive aids and flavor enhancers. Spices such as coriander, cumin, turmeric, black and white pepper, curry, fenugreek, fennel, cinnamon, clove, cardamom, and saffron are valued not only in Ayurvedic medicine, but in many culinary traditions. Cayenne, jalapeno, and other chili peppers are eaten daily by one third of the world's population, and not just in Central, and South America. However, some don't take well to hot spices such as cayenne, jalapeno, or chili, so I would recommend those folks explore other options to increase digestive fire. Adding the right amount and kind of spice to your food will significantly increase your digestive capacity.

Lemon Water. Mix approximately nine parts of distilled water to one part of fresh squeezed lemon juice. Take two to four ounces of the mixture once in the morning and once at night. This helps give the liver the substances it needs to digest food.[4] (Using a straw may help conserve tooth enamel for sensitive people.)

Digestive Aids

Digestive enzymes are produced by our glands. Each part of our digestive tract makes its own set of enzymes: the salivary glands, the stomach, the small intestine, and the pancreas.[5] The pancreas has two functions: to help digest food and to regulate blood sugar. Damage to the sugar-handling mechanism of the pancreas (resulting in diabetes) is often associated with gum disease. One particular type of digestive enzymes that I found effective are proteolytic enzymes made from freeze-dried pig pancreas. These support diminished pancreatic function. Some examples of proteolytic enzymes or systemic enzymes are freeze-dried pig pancreas or *Wobenzym® N.*

Another type of digestive enzymes can be taken with meals and these are the ones most often found in health food stores. These may be also helpful for some readers, but I do not have a particular brand recommendation right now.

Ox bile was a historically-prescribed remedy for gum disease.[6] A small capsule was taken just after a meal to aid the digestion of fat. If the ox bile supplement does not produce discomfort or diarrhea after taking it with food, then you likely have bile insufficiency. Ox bile supports the function of the gall bladder. At this time not enough information is available to recommend a brand or specific dosages.

Hydrochloric acid is another common remedy for digestive problems. The stomach must produce ample amounts of highly acidic digestive fluids to both digest food and destroy pathogens in the stomach. Paradoxically, it is actually too little hydrochloric acid rather than too much that leads to acid reflux disorder.

Note: Enzymes, ox bile, and hydrochloric acid are digestive crutches best taken with the guidance and supervision of a holistically-oriented physician or other holistic licensed health care provider. While they are useful, it is always best to address the root cause of the deficiencies.

Historical Remedies to Support Digestion

Digestive problems are often caused by toxic substances or cellular waste that is stuck in the excretion pathways of the body. Therefore, improving digestion permanently often requires strategies to give the body good nutrition, as well as open the clogged elimination pathways. The historical approach to cleansing clogged channels as it related to gum disease in the U.S. and Europe was through probiotics, exercise, sweating, and massage.[7]

Exercise can help clear clogged channels in the body through sweating, creating motion in bodily fluids, and from helping use up and excrete biological substances.[8] Find a type of exercise that feels good and is enjoyable and do it consistently. Keep in mind that highly intense forms of exercise put the body under stress and increase nutritional demands, so if you exercise a lot you need to eat plenty of calories.

Sweating through saunas or sweat lodges is an ancient tradition of cleansing practiced in many places around the world. Sweating deeply cleanses some of the channels in the body.[9]

Therapeutic massage can open up channels in the body, free up physical restrictions, and help you attain a higher level of health.[10] There are many types of massage and techniques. I do not have a recommendation of one being better than another, but allowing your body to receive support, to overcome stagnation by increasing circulation, to relax, and to release tension will surely aid your healing process. Based in part on Ayurvedic cleansing, one can do an oil massage to bring toxins closer to the surface of the body then immediately follow it by sweating. This can be an excellent way to detoxify. We personally do these at home. One can even do a self oil massage, and then sweat in a portable sauna.

Intermediate Cleansing Suggestions

Many people will not regain their digestive powers without a deeper cleansing of the body. On my website **curegumdisease.com/cleansing**, I have provided detailed information with additional links and resources to help you understand cleansing options. They are briefly summarized here.

Coffee Enemas

Coffee Enemas are an effective way for cleansing the bowels, liver, and gall bladder. Often digestion is sluggish because the liver is congestion and the bile is not flowing freely. Consistent coffee enemas are one method to resolve this problem. Enemas used to be recommended by many doctors and were a standard medical procedure described in older medical reference manuals. To perform a coffee enema, boil one quart of purified water with two tablespoons of organic coffee for five minutes. Cool to a comfortable temperature and proceed with enema. Try to retain the coffee for at least ten minutes.

Fasting and Juice Fasting

Fasting gives time for the body to rest and clear out any accumulated waste. There are many ways to fast, although if you are underweight, fasting might not be the best way for you to get healthy because fasting depletes minerals from the body.

A water-only fast can be done for one to three days. Juice fasting can be carried out for a longer period of time. This is best done primarily with vegetable juices, because fruit juices are generally too sweet and can cause blood sugar problems. Fasting can be combined with enemas, such as with the Dr. Bernard Jensen (1908 – 2001) tissue cleansing program. There are also many types of herbal cleansing systems on the market. Fasts are best done under the care and supervision of your health professional.

Raw Milk Cleanse

Raw milk cleansing used to be a standard procedure. Dr. J. R. Crewe, of the Mayo Foundation, supervised many patients' milk fasts with excellent results.[11] There are many ways to cleanse with raw milk. One method involves a short introductory water fast and then living only on raw cow or goat's milk for a period of days or weeks. It can begin with one ounce of room temperature fresh cow milk taken seven times daily. The dosages increase incrementally every day. By the thirteenth day one is consuming ten-ounce servings of milk twelve times per day. This can be continued under the supervision of a health practitioner for forty days. The same cleanse can be carried out with real buttermilk—the liquid of freshly churned butter, specifically butter made from yogurt. This is done by mixing ¾ cup of fresh buttermilk with ¼ cup of water.[12] Note that this fast will only work with raw milk from healthy animals eating their natural diet. This type of cleanse can help gum disease patients in two ways. First, it can clean the toxic acidic waste from the body and enhance functioning of the digestive system, and second, it is a high calcium diet, and calcium is essential to reversing gum disease. More information is found at: realmilk.com/health/milk-cure/

Broth and Yogurt Cleanse

This is accomplished by consuming one cup of fresh goat yogurt morning and night. For other meals, one consumes a rich chicken broth with chicken meat and plenty of vegetables, including plenty of zucchini.

Liver and Gall Bladder Flush

The purpose of this cleanse is to expel deposits and stones from the liver and gall bladder. This cleanse involves drinking apple juice to loosen gall stones, taking Epsom salts to open up elimination channels, and then taking a mixture of olive oil and lemon juice to release bile out of the liver. There are many ways to perform this cleanse, some more aggressive than others.

Again, learn more about all of these methods at: curegumdisease.com/cleansing

Ayurvedic Cleansing with Panchakarma

Traditional Ayurvedic medicine relies on a complex system of cleansing called Panchakarma that includes oil massages, herbs, a restricted diet of mung beans and rice (kitchari), steam baths, enemas, and medicated ghee. Panchakarma can be done at home, but if you can afford it, getting help from an Ayurvedic health professional will probably lead to much better results. The fee for the complete therapy can add up, however, with full treatment regimens you will probably feel a lot better. Many people who have done Panchakarma recommend it, but finding a good practitioner is important for optimal results and comfort.

Traditional Chinese Medicine offers herbal formulas, acupuncture, and other remedies for poor digestion, balancing body chemistry, and strengthening weak or deficient systems of the body. Because the traditional system is safe, effective, generally affordable, and practitioners are easy to find near most urban centers, it is worth looking into if you want more support for your digestion or help with gum disease.

Little Known but Important Causes of Poor Digestion

There are some folks who have tried many alternative health practitioners, eat a very clean diet with nutrient-dense foods, and still fail to recover from health problems like tooth decay and gum disease. This brief section is to summarize some other factors that can cause the chronic digestive distress. These are problems that even few natural health care providers know about or can diagnose properly.

One way to try to discover what is making you unhealthy is to try to recall any event in your life after which your body changed from being healthy to beset with illness. Understanding the event that caused illness is a key toward seeking the right treatment to unwind the problem.

There are a few conditions that can commonly cause problems in the body that will affect digestion and assimilation.

1. **Hidden infections** can occur at the site of root canals or tooth extractions. These are discussed in chapter nine on dentistry. The hidden infection leaks toxic substances throughout the body. The body tries to excrete these substances, possibly through the digestive tract, causing feelings of weakness and nausea. The solution is to locate and heal the hidden infections or boost the body's immunity enough to deal with them.
2. **Head injuries** are caused by car accidents and other accidents, especially during the growing years. Orthodontic work during the growing years is also like a head injury, although in slow motion. Jaw surgery can freeze up the cranial motion and significantly interfere with digestion and also create sites of chronic infection. Head injuries restrict the movement of cranial-sacral fluid and may impinge upon the normal functioning of the nervous system. As a result, the body becomes stuck in sympathetic nervous system overdrive. It cannot relax and no matter what is tried, it is difficult to rest, digest, and sleep well. The solution is getting cranial-sacral work or other bodywork to help heal and release the head injury.
3. **Surgeries** can be especially traumatizing to the body. Removing the appendix, gall bladder, uterus, or prostate, as well as Cesarean section surgery, are all substantially shocking to the body. If you notice a sudden change in bodily functioning after these sorts of surgical procedures, then your system may have developed various problems associated with the surgery. This includes remnants of antibiotics or anesthesia in the spinal fluid, incomplete wound healing causing a hidden infection in the body (you can palpate the area to see if it is very tender as one sign of an infection), and problematic scar tissue or adhesions from incisions that freeze up the natural pulsations and motility of the digestive organs. Practitioners who work deeply with the body on scar tissue, organ manipulation, and so forth might be able to help with some of these conditions.
4. **Emotional trauma** that is unresolved can cause digestive problems. When a violation or wound happens to us, our tendency is to hide the very shameful feelings associated with the violation. It is as if a part of us "swallows" our pain and closes it off. Trying to escape the past or trying to forget about a painful or shocking event in life does not mean the problem is resolved. Instead, the event lives on in

both our psyche and our physical tissues. The way to heal this is to start talking about the unresolved feelings to someone who is able to listen to them such as a trusted friend or a holistically-oriented psychologist.

5. **Sleep.** When you eat well, and detoxify, your body needs time to repair and rebuild. This happens during sleep. Restful sleep is the experience of being deeply relaxed, and going into a healing state of stillness. With restful sleep, one wakes up refreshed. Not restful sleep is stressful, and usually results in difficulty in waking. When it is time to wake up, your body feels unhappy, and it wants to sleep more, but feels unable to rest. Of course you should give yourself the gift of time to rest and relax. Make sure you give your body enough hours to sleep so that you have time to heal. Even with enough time, some people often do not sleep well. A glass of warm grass-fed milk before bed can help. If you have had orthodontic braces or headgear in the past, then you may suffer from some form of sleep apnea. This is when the body does not get enough oxygen during sleep, and thus it does not relax or heal properly. The temporary solution for sleep apnea is a sleep apnea night guard to help with proper jaw position (some dentists specialize in these). While it is hard to pinpoint what your sleep problem could be, just make sure you are sleeping well and enough, and if you are not sleeping enough, this could be a significant hindrance to your health. Also make sure to turn off Wi-Fi at night, and preferably turn off the electric power to your bedroom, so that you have a more restful space. Also keep electronic devices and cell phones that are on well away from you at night.
6. **Heavy Metal Poisoning** – Heavy metal poisoning, along with other types of poisoning from toxins in the environment or from food can underlie many digestive problems and problems of acidity and inflammation in the body. In the previous chapter you learned about the significant connection between mercury poisoning and gum disease. Often the heavy metals are hidden in deep layers of the body tissue, and for some people, they do not just come out on their own. If you suspect heavy metal poisoning, it can be useful to find an alternative medicine practitioner who specializes in heavy metal detoxification. In general, natural heavy metal detoxification requires:

    - ☐ Cleansing and supporting the liver function
    - ☐ Opening excretion channels
    - ☐ Binding toxins in the intestine
    - ☐ Supporting the body with specific nutrients

Vegetables for Vitamins, Minerals, and Balance

We are told to cook our meat, chicken, or fish completely to avoid harmful bacteria. Meanwhile, many health-oriented authorities recommend we eat vegetables raw to preserve nutrients and enzymes. But uncooked vegetables contain a host of plant toxins including enzyme inhibitors, oxalates, saponins, and lectins.[13] Besides a few exceptions such as lettuce or cucumber, raw vegetables are in fact harder to digest than cooked vegetables. Only people with strong digestive powers can thrive on uncooked vegetables.[14] For the rest of us, we need heat or fermentation to break down the vegetable cellulose. Unless you have very strong digestive fires, eating a great deal of raw vegetables is not a healthy practice because of the plant toxins and potentially irritating raw plant fiber.[15] Vegetables should be prepared so that they are easy to digest and assimilate, as well as taste good. Vegetables cooked soft with plenty of butter or other good fats are the best option for many people on a healing journey.

If you visit a farm you can watch goats or cows madly salivate over grass. I have noticed that reaction does not occur with humans. That is because we are not made to eat too many uncooked, raw, fibrous vegetables. Raw vegetables can irritate the intestinal lining especially if the lining is already inflamed. Cooked vegetables and fruits have their cellulose broken down so they are easier for us to digest. To me, a soft cooked piece of broccoli with some butter or cheese is much easier to digest than a piece of raw crunchy broccoli. When vegetables are juiced, the cellulose is removed mechanically and the nutrients are free to be assimilated.

Dark, leafy-green vegetables need to be eaten cooked, as the nutrients are released through cooking.[16] The bottom line is to prepare your vegetables in ways that promote digestibility and good taste. While raw vegetables serve some people well as part of a temporary cleanse therapy, do not force yourself to eat raw vegetables every day unless you truly enjoy them.

Fermentation is a form of processing the vegetable that makes it easier to digest. Do avail yourself to fermented vegetables.

Alkalize Your Body and Live

People with healthy digestive systems are not likely to produce digestive toxins and their bodies will not likely become inflamed or acidic from eating lots of fatty or rich foods like bacon and red meat. However, people with compromised digestive systems can easily become overly acidic from the overeating of red meat, shellfish, and animal fats such as lard and tallow. The solution is to avoid and limit acidifying foods during the healing period in which you are reducing inflammation in your body.

Since every reader is different, not all readers need to become that much more alkaline. People with type 1 gum disease as described in chapter three, which represent about 75 percent of severe gum disease cases, need to become more alkaline due to underlying toxicities and physiological imbalances. But 23 percent of gum disease cases, as with type 2 gum disease, may be alkaline enough, or may just need to become only slightly more alkaline. Most readers who fall into this category are moderately healthy, and are simply just not eating enough of the right foods. It is possible to become too alkaline if one goes overboard on juicing and cleansing when one needs to build instead of cleanse.

Alkalizing Your Body with Vegetables

Juicing saves lives. Raw vegetable juice has enzymes, vitamins, and minerals that help remove stagnant plaque from the body, clear lymphatic congestion, and tone the liver.[17] It can help remove heavy metals and balance the acidity in the body. I personally have been juicing regularly for about eight years, and no matter how many times I have taken a break, or have given up due to the time it takes, I always return to it because of how good I feel from juicing. If you choose the right vegetables that are not too sweet and not too hard on the body, juicing removes the fibrous irritants by removing the indigestible vegetable fiber.

Exercise caution when juicing and making green smoothies (smoothies made by blending vegetables). Not all vegetables are safe for everyone to regularly consume raw in large quantities. Vegetables that are safer for juicing over the long run are organic zucchini, string beans, cilantro, parsley, cucumber, and celery. Carrot and beet juices are okay to drink but extremely sweet, thus contributing to blood sugar imbalances.

Green smoothies are a popular trend, but take care. Often entire raw green vegetables that contain plant toxins in their raw form are used like spinach, kale, broccoli, asparagus, cabbage, chard, and other dense leafy greens. For the short term, this may not be a problem, but for the long run it has caused toxicity problems and illness for some people. Furthermore, people who use too much fruit to make green smoothies palatable will experience calcium losses over time because of the high sugar intake.

I have experienced the cleansing power of raw vegetables, and they seem to balance well with a diet that also includes healthy animal fats, calcium from grass-fed dairy products, and healthy animal protein.

I drink juices between meals and that is what some other health experts also recommend. So I am not advising an exclusive juice diet, but rather, drinking juices in between your nourishing meals to alkalize the body, to enhance digestion, and to give your tissues enzymes and minerals.

Alkalizing Vegetable Juice Recipe

Feel free to change this recipe to your liking. All ingredients should be organic.

4 medium zucchinis
2 cucumbers
1 bunch of celery stalks
2 bunches of fresh cilantro
2 bunches fresh parsley
Optional - ½ green apple for flavor
Optional – Stir up to ¾ cup of raw cream into the finished juice
Juice the ingredients with a juicer and enjoy.

I use a Green Star twin gear juicer. It is more work than other types of juicers because of cutting and prepping the vegetables, but it extracts more juice at lower speeds than most juicers. Centrifuge juicers are acceptable to me, but other health experts say they are too damaging to the vegetables because of their high speed. Press juicers are used in cancer therapy because the cellular structure of the mineral and vitamin-rich vegetable fluid remains the most intact, so a press juicer will also produce fine juice for you. Mixing the finished juice with a small amount of raw honey helps prolong its freshness.[18] Mixing the juice with raw cow cream or raw coconut cream, the cream of a juiced coconut (not coconut milk), gives the juice an entirely different restorative attribute as the fat helps the body assimilate the minerals in the juice and it tastes quite good. Drinking juice is a much better alternative to drinking coffee in the morning because it is energizing and gives the body vitamins and minerals from whole foods.

Dr. Bieler's Alkalizing Vegetable Soup

This is the original healing soup of Dr. Henry Bieler (1893 – 1975), author of *Food is Your Best Medicine*, and will help alkalize your body and nourish your glands.

1 pound of string beans, ends removed
2 pounds zucchini, chopped
1 handful of curly parsley
Enough water to cover your veggies

Add all ingredients to rapidly boiling water and boil for ten to fifteen minutes, or until a fork easily pierces the zucchini skin. Purée using the cooking water (it is important to use this water as it contains vitamins and minerals) and make the soup to the consistency you desire.

This specific recipe is designed for healing when the body is ill. Dr. Bieler sometimes prescribed a short fast (twenty-four hours or so) with this soup. Feel free to modify this recipe by adding all kinds of different vegetables to make a soup to suit your personal needs. These mineral-rich vegetables can be combined with ginger and chicken stock to make a heavenly soup, although it may be somewhat less alkalizing.

Dried Greens and Dried Wheatgrass

For people who want to alkalize but are unable or unwilling to make juice or green smoothies, you can learn more about high-quality dried wheatgrass and dried green powder supplements that support alkalizing the body at: curegumdisease.com/alkalize

Cure Gum Disease with Lifestyle Changes

Healing gum disease for many people is not just about changing what one puts in our body; it is about changing how one views themselves, life, and others. When we view the world from a negative place, we are disconnected, frozen, and inwardly stagnant. Releasing this inner stagnation brings us to life. I have some suggestions to help you change your focus and change the way you live and see the world.

First, one needs to align oneself with a vision or picture of perfect health. Align yourself with the Divine Health of the Creator, or, if you prefer, the Divine Health of the Universe.

You are a perfect being of creation. There is a template, plan, or a set of unseen rules you can follow to make yourself healthy. Several times per day, visualize, feel, or meditate upon your health.

1. Take a deep breath
2. Align yourself with an image of health.
3. Feel it in your body.
4. Feel your body without gum disease.
5. Feel your body radiating with health, aliveness, hope, goodness, and vitality.

Every day is precious. But when we are ill, every day can easily feel miserable and like a defeat. Use your mind, feelings, and willpower to change your destiny. Visualize your body with healthy digestion and healthy gums.

Support Your Body's Detoxification

Get out and move. Stop spending life just watching movies, or television, reading all the time, playing video games, or browsing the Internet. Find a type of movement you enjoy and do it at least twice a week. Choose at least one type of movement and give it a try. A few examples of movement are long walks, yoga, tai chi, dance, fitness class at the gym, sports, and swimming. Movement moves the fluids of your body and increases the speed of recovery and repair, and it helps you feel good by boosting your mood.

Follow Your Dreams

Life can be fleeting and may end at any moment. Dare to do something different. Follow a forgotten dream. Reconnect with an estranged relative or friend. Dare to live to the fullest. Make the most of your life. Make a change in the world. Do something kind for someone else. Share a meal. Say thank you. Practice gratitude. Stop putting off your life. Start living!

Healing Your Environment

As I've previously stated in the last chapter and in this one, I highly recommend that you reduce electromagnetic field exposure (EMFs) by eliminating Wi-Fi completely in your house. We use wired Internet. It may not be the most convenient option, but it helps protect the nervous system. If you cannot always turn off Wi-Fi, minimize its use and turn it off at night.

You can also further reduce your EMF exposure by:

- ☐ Turning off the power to your bedroom at night at the circuit breaker, or at least keeping electric devices away from your bed.
- ☐ Use a headset with your cell phone and keep your cell phone physically away from your body. Use an anti-radiation shield for your cell phone such as a Pong™ case. Minimize cell phone use. Use a corded landline phone instead of a cordless phone.

Get out in the fresh air and practice some deep breathing at a park with trees every day. Walk barefoot where possible.

Getting Support

Have someone your trust read this book so they can help you out. Tell them your struggles and fears. Enlist them to help you to locate and eat the right kinds of foods. Have them check in with you as you follow the protocols you have chosen to invest your energy in. Just make sure that the person you choose for your support system is open minded enough to be supportive of whatever you want to try. Conversely, if you have people in your life who are bringing you down, doubting your every move, and trying to get you to submit to things you know are wrong for you, be brave and tell them where you stand and ask them to stop.

There are also many professionals in allied fields that can help you with your journey to health, including therapies such as cranial sacral (upledger.com), acupuncture, chiropractic care, massage, lymph drainage, functional medicine, nutritional support, and more.

Now that you have some idea on how to increase your health and your digestive strength, let's look at what to eat to stop gum disease naturally.

Chapter 7 Summary – Good Digestion Is Necessary for Healthy Gums

- ☐ Disease begins in the digestive tract.
- ☐ Many people with gum disease do not digest food well. The symptoms of poor digestion include gas, constipation, diarrhea, burping, burning sensations, vomiting, indigestion, bloating, and pain after eating.
- ☐ Incomplete digestion, putrefaction, poisoning, and electromagnetic field poison may be contributing to your gum disease.
- ☐ Good digestion is essential to gum health. Digestive aids include: organic apple cider vinegar, spices, lemon water, digestive enzymes, ox bile, and hydrochloric acid.

- □ Procedures to rejuvenate digestion and support health include: exercise, sweating, therapeutic massage, coffee enemas, fasting, juice fasting, raw milk cleansing, liver and gall bladder flushes, Ayurvedic cleansing with Panchakarma, and traditional Chinese Medicine.
- □ Little known but important causes of poor digestion may be hidden infections, head injuries, surgeries, emotional trauma, lack of sleep, and heavy metal poisoning.
- □ Vegetables need to be prepared well to support digestion and the balancing of body chemistry. Raw vegetables can irritate the intestinal lining, especially if the lining is already inflamed. Cooked vegetables and fruits have their cellulose broken down so they are easier for us to digest. Vegetable juicing with the focus on organic zucchini, string beans, cilantro, parsley, cucumber, and celery is recommended as an addition to one's diet, between meals. Fruit juicing can lead to a loss of calcium over time due to the high sugar intake. Vegetable soup such as Dr. Beiler's is also recommended.
- □ Lifestyle changes will help cure gum disease. Visualizing ourselves as healthy, meditation, movement, nourishing activities, pursuing our dreams, healing our environments, reducing our exposure to EMFs, and getting emotional support are all recommended.

8 Cure Gum Disease Naturally with A, B, C, D, and K

Healing gum disease nutritionally requires restoring the missing fat-soluble vitamins and minerals to our diet. This chapter synthesizes all the information from the entire book into guidelines and protocols that you can incorporate into your own life.

Curing Gum Disease Is *Almost* as easy as A, B, C, D, and K

Here are some of the principal vitamins that are vital to incorporate into your gum healing diet along with some alphabetically listed reminders of key concepts in oral health.

A – Vitamin A prevents teeth from becoming loose by nourishing and strengthening the periodontal ligament and minimizing gum tissue irritation.

A – Acidity is typical in type 1 gum disease as discussed in chapter seven. Excessive acidity needs to be eliminated so that the body chemistry can be restored to health and balance. This can usually be accomplished through a program of detoxification and by consumption of greens.

B – B vitamins are abundant in liver, wild fish, pastured meats. and poultry.

B – Bone broth, collagen, or a cartilage-rich supplement will help with bone strengthening and nutrient absorption.

C – Vitamin C is crucial for gum health and reduction and mitigation of toxicities in the body.

C – Calories count. People who deprive themselves of food will not get the nourishment they need. On the other hand, there are plenty of malnourished people who consume excess calories in overly processed and denatured foods that cannot nourish their bodies. Choose nutrient-dense foods that will satisfy your hunger.

D – Vitamin D from sources such as real cod liver oil is required for calcium and mineral metabolism.

D – Everyone is different and unique. Not everyone needs the same thing nutritionally. Listen to your body and if you can, find a way to test supplements or dietary ideas with the bio-energetic system of your body using applied kinesiology, muscle testing, dowsing, cranial rhythm, or other intuitive faculties.

K – Vitamin "K2"/Activator X. This fat-soluble vitamin matrix helps rebuild and strengthen your periodontium. Again, for the sake of gum healing, I only recommend foods rich in activator X/"K2" that are from wild or humanely raised animal foods such as fish eggs, pastured butter, cultured grass-fed dairy or cheese, and very likely in bone marrow and organs like brain, kidney, tripe, spleen, pancreas, heart, sweetbreads, animal blood, and lungs.

K – Kelp, a small amount of kelp is excellent for trace mineral support along with the highly essential iodine. The trace minerals in kelp synergize with the fat-soluble vitamins.[1]

The diet outline below involves several important aspects to heal gum disease. This outline will help you understand from an overview what foods need to be added to or removed from your diet in a way that is flexible and affirming to your dietary needs.

1. Add fat-soluble vitamins A, D, and Activator X/"K2" to your diet.
2. Consume adequate portions of protein with every meal to help maintain balanced blood sugar.
3. Avoid or reduce modern denatured foods.
4. In the case of type 1 gum disease, alkalizing foods will be very helpful.
5. Eat mineral-dense foods like broth, dairy products, kelp, organs, and organic vegetables.

Healthy Fats, Proteins, and Carbs

Healthy Fats Are Essential for Gum Health

Now that the myth that saturated fat is unhealthy has been thoroughly and completely debunked, feel free to enjoy butter, red meat, eggs, organ meats, coconut oil, and whole milk.[2] Even the Harvard School of Public Health declares, "It's time to end the low-fat myth."[3]

How much fat each person needs varies. When fat is not properly metabolized, it can cause inflammation. Some signs of poor fat digestion are inflamed joints, feeling overly full, lethargic, or depressed after eating fatty foods. If you have these symptoms, your liver likely needs to be cleared through detoxification and / or supported with bile and / or pancreas supplements while moderating fat consumption until the problem is solved.

The fat-soluble vitamins A, D, and activator X/"K2" *are absolutely essential* to revitalizing the periodontium and halting gum disease. Here are my suggestions to obtain these essential vitamins:

1. Satisfy your appetite for fat and never deprive yourself of it.
2. Consume plenty of butter or ghee, preferably cultured and from pastured cows.
3. Listen to your body, experiment, and know that your fat needs can change from day to day.
4. Vitamin D is absolutely essential to healing gum disease. Consume high vitamin D-rich foods and/or supplement it with real cod liver oil or skate liver oil.

I believe animal fats are healthy and surely most of our bodies crave them. But some people have gum disease and are eating lots of animal fats and not improving because the high fat foods are not being metabolized. This can happen because certain fats cause imbalances in people who have fat-metabolism problems. If you find you are not getting better, then consider removing foods that could be a problem, including **bacon, lamb, fatty beef, nuts and nut oils like peanuts and sunflower, doughnuts, chocolate, olives, and potato chips.**[4]

Protein for Your Teeth and Gums

The alveolar bone is comprised of five percent protein. Eating high quality protein in the form of grass-fed meat or wild game or fish will give gum tissue the high quality building blocks it needs. Good quality muscle meat (chicken, beef, fish, etc.) contains phosphorus, amino acids, and other minerals that can build healthy bones. Homemade bone broth, made from cartilage and bones, is rich in the conditionally essential amino acids proline and glycine, which are keys to the healthy collagen we need for teeth, gums, and the alveolar bone.

Organs and glands provide the missing fat-soluble vitamins and cofactors in our modern diet. In many countries across the world, people still consume organ meats and glands regularly. In our modern western culture, this habit has been lost, and as a result our growing boys and girls often develop poor facial structures and do not build strong bodies. Over a long period of time, without these nutrients from animal sources, our bodies become more susceptible to disease. The evidence of traditional peoples from around the world suggests "nose to tail eating" is the key to a healthy body and healthy mouth. Consuming many parts of the animal is an essential component to restoring your health and balancing your blood chemistry. If you do not regularly consume a wide variety of organ meats, consider adding them to your diet and/or buying an organ and gland supplement such as the one available at traditionalfoods.org.

Enhancing Protein Assimilation

The cooking methods mentioned here can increase your ability to safely digest and utilize proteins as well as improve the flavor of food and increase your pleasure in eating. Because proteins are body builders, proper cooking will increase protein assimilation and help stop gum disease.

Barbecue – Grill your food on wood coals. This adds a wonderful flavor and a juicy texture to your food. Commercially prepared charcoal with chemicals added can make food toxic, but real wood, or real wood coals without added chemicals for barbecues leaves your proteins juicy and flavorful.[5] Foods cooked on a grill taste addictively good. Marinating the meat beforehand for at least several hours can reduce potentially carcinogenic compounds from forming.[6]

Rare – A well-done steak generally does not taste as good as one cooked to medium rare or rare. Beef, lamb, and tuna all taste great seared but not fully cooked.

Stews – Eating fully cooked proteins with a gelatin-rich broth as stew or with gravy enhances your body's ability to digest the protein. Cooked protein repels digestive juices in our stomachs. But mixing cooked protein with a gelatin-rich broth that attracts digestive juices helps the body digest the whole meal well.[7]

Raw – Many cuisines feature raw protein foods, although they often go unnoticed. Body builders favor raw eggs in smoothies. Other common raw foods are steak tartare, sushi, sashimi, cheese, and oysters. Some people have no problem eating animal foods raw; I have done it countless times. Other people prefer to freeze or marinate animal proteins before they consume them raw to destroy possible pathogens or potential parasites. Raw protein can be very easy to digest because it attracts digestive juices in the stomach.[8]

No-Heat "Cooking" – We have cured and fermented raw meats available in our culture. Salami, cold smoked salmon, and corned beef are a few examples. Although many store-bought versions are cooked, some artisanally-produced versions are not. Ceviche is an example of acid from lemon or lime juice "cooking" the food (raw fish) while it marinates. These types of no-heat cooking methods make protein easy to digest and taste good.

The Healthy Amount of Protein to Consume

People's protein needs vary according to age, weight, climate, season, level of physical activity, and their digestive ability. It is important to listen to your body and feel what your protein needs are first and foremost. I provide you with two methods to measure and help you tune in to or sense your own daily protein needs below:

Method 1, Moderate Protein – This is based on the work of Dr. Melvin Page. These are amounts based on your ideal body weight, not your current body weight.

100 pounds: 6.5 ounces of protein
120 pounds: 8 ounces of protein
150 pounds: 10 ounces of protein
180 pounds: 12 ounces of protein

For other weights, calculate 1 ounce of protein per 15 pounds of ideal body weight.

Method 2, Higher Protein – Men consume two palm-size portions of protein per meal, and women one-palm size portion.[9]

Reduce Stress with Adequate Calories and Adequate Carbohydrates

In reviewing cases of people who suffer from gum disease, I found two frequent dietary patterns: calorie restriction and carbohydrate restriction. In order to heal gum disease, do not unnecessarily restrict calories and be sure to eat enough to satisfy your appetite. And if your digestion allows, consume as much carbohydrate foods as you need to fuel your movement level.

Calorie restriction occurs more often with women than men because of body image issues and self-imposed pressures. People who severely cut calories to become fashionably thin can send their bodies into starvation mode. This, in turn, engages the demineralization process, leading to deficiencies of calcium, phosphorous, and trace minerals, and eventually to type II gum disease. When people fail to eat enough food, the body pulls minerals out of its reserves in the bones and fat out of the marrow. Pregnancy, breastfeeding, and strenuous exercise severely deplete the body **when calorie intake is not sufficient,** resulting in the common symptoms of gum disease or tooth decay and bone loss in relation to pregnancy.

To maintain excellent health, it is essential to stay well nourished, eat regularly, and stay fit. Good looks do not depend on weight alone but on muscle tone, good hormonal function, and bone density. Given that muscle weighs more than fat, and mineral density often means stronger bones, it's possible to look slimmer and yet gain weight. Eating plenty for many people creates the best chances to get adequate energy, minerals, and vitamins from our diet to be healthy.

Many people today endorse a low-carb diet rich in fat and protein. Following such a diet may initially feel good and help lose unwanted pounds, but any overly restrictive diet tends to fail after the honeymoon phase.[10] What I have noticed when I restrict carbohydrates is that my calorie consumption significantly drops, and my enjoyment of proteins and fats significantly decreases. For me, carbohydrates mixed with fats or proteins make a happy marriage. Some of the foods people crave most are such calorie-rich combinations. Think of pie and ice cream (carbs and fat), a cheeseburger (carbs, fat, and protein), or grilled cheese sandwich (carbs, protein, and fat). If carbohydrate restriction is improving your body chemistry and you continue to feel healthy while cutting carbohydrates, then there is no need to stop. However, some signs that a low-carb diet is not working are moodiness, loss of sex drive, hair loss, increased fat and decreased muscle, low energy levels, feeling cold, and having cold hands and feet.[11]

An abundance of research indicates that a moderate or higher carbohydrate diet helps support thyroid function, and that an absence of carbohydrates reduces thyroid function. Carbohydrate research also shows that moderate and higher carbohydrate diets are not associated with weight gain and that eating carbohydrates helps balance hormonal levels.[12] The bottom line is that for many readers avoiding or restricting carbohydrates for too long may not promote health and in fact may cause harm.

Grain-Free Carbohydrates and Dietary Healing

Some people experience great healing when consuming large amounts of grass-fed dairy products including yogurt, kefir, and/or milk. Plenty of these foods provide adequate nutrient-dense carbohydrates (along with protein and fat) without the need for starches or grains.

Clarifying Macronutrients

There are many well-known authors and books that provide ample evidence for the argument that carbohydrates make us fat and that we should avoid them.[13] It is important to understand that most authors advocating such a position are ultimately writing from their own personal experience (as I am here as well.) Some people do fantastically well on a high-fat, low-carb diet and so they promote it. But for many people a balanced diet does not avoid any food major category (protein, carbohydrates, or fat). If you can get enough calories on a high-fat diet and your gum disease goes into remission, by all means do so. In general, I think readers with significant gum disease will ultimately benefit from a balanced approach. I have found that a balanced approach allows me to consume the most calories and feel the best. But try not to get stuck in any dietary paradigms. Think for yourself. Listen to your body. You are your own master. Trust your cravings and instincts and find ways to nurture yourself with food and enjoy eating. And if one dietary paradigm does not work for you, then simply try something else.

Four Dietary Programs Designed for Different Needs

I am sharing four dietary programs to address the concerns of four main types of readers. I suggest reading all of the programs because there is minimal repetition and each program has something that can be learned from it.

General dietary guidelines are for people who want to get healthy on a well-rounded diet. You are interested in eating well, but do not feel the need at this time to do more serious body chemistry balancing. It allows for a wide variety of food while giving specific instructions on how to remineralize and restore the body.

The **balancing diet** program is more restrictive and made for people who are avoiding gluten, grains, and possibly dairy products. It is designed to help balance body chemistry more than the first program due to the avoidance of high carbohydrate foods. It is possible to start with this body chemistry balancing program and then switch to the **general program** after a few weeks.

The **simple** program is for readers who feel overwhelmed or just want to try something different without making big changes. The results may not be as good, but making some changes is better than none at all.

And this book would not be complete without an **extreme program**. I know some of my readers want to truly heal their body with only foods. So I offer a complete, raw animal and plant food diet outline.

Three Dietary Essentials for Creating Your Healing Diet

1. **Trust yourself and your instincts:** As the master of your destiny, only you can walk the straight and narrow path toward health. Health requires internalizing dietary principles, but at the same time, trusting your gut, or your instincts. Listen to your taste buds and follow those inner signals. Do not get stuck in rigid dogmas; rather, relax and nourish yourself. In the end, the best choices come from a deep knowing within, and my purpose in this book is to create a framework to help you connect with that knowing.
2. **Connect with your food heritage:** Each one of us comes from generations of people who knew how to be healthy and how to live in some degree of harmony with the land. In previous generations, we learned what to eat and what was healthy from our parents, grandparents, and extended family. Only in relatively recent times, in just the last century, has the generational/ancestral food knowledge become lost and supplanted. No longer do we learn about healthy foods from our family; we now learn from public schools, advertisements, television, and the government. Unfortunately maleficent forces have influenced our communal food knowledge and the wise food choices of our familiar lineage have been supplanted by unwholesome and harmful substitutes. Generally foods from our own ancestral lineage work best for us. Talk to your parents, grandparents, or other relatives to help reconnect with traditional foods ways. Also think back to family meals during childhood or special occasions when traditional foods of your family's heritage were eaten. Typically these foods will be most easily absorbed and digested by you.
3. **Fermented dairy products from pastured animals:** Whole milk can be harder to digest in its refrigerated, sweet form. Traditional cultures across the world ferment milk to predigest casein and lactose. Fermented dairy products can be very healing and medicinal. Cheese, yogurt, and kefir are a few examples of fermented/cultured dairy products.[14]

Cure Gum Disease General Dietary Guidelines

6+ ounces of protein per day from healthy animal sources such as pasture-raised chicken, turkey, pork, beef, and /or from wild fish such as tuna, salmon, and sardines.

Calcium: Most people need between 1,200mg (1.2g) to 2,000mg (2g) grams of calcium per day; the average person needs about 1.5g. Excellent sources of calcium include dairy products from pastured goats, sheep, cows, mares, camels, or from whole bone meal.

With Dairy

2-4 cups of raw dairy products per day (600mg to 1,200mg of calcium) in the form of milk, kefir, whey, yogurt, clabber, or buttermilk. You can substitute about two ounces of cheese for every cup of fluid milk.

1-2 ounces of raw cheese (200-400mg of calcium).

Without Dairy

1½ -3 teaspoons *Bone Marrow & Cartilage Calcium* (600mg – 1,200mg of calcium).

½ - 1 teaspoon *Whole Bone Calcium* (770mg – 1,440mg of calcium).

Healthy Fat – Activator X/"K2"

½ - 3 tablespoons of grass-fed butter or ghee, cultured preferred

Alkalizing Factors

Choose at least one of the following per day:

4-8 ounces of fresh green veggie juice, 2-4 times per day in between meals.

Plenty of cooked vegetables such as, but not limited to, beet greens, kale, chard, zucchini, broccoli, celery, and string beans.

Least preferred option: green juice powder (sweetener-free) 2-4 times per day (suggestions at: curegumdisease.com/alkalize).

Vitamin C

¼ – 2 teaspoons of *High Vitamin C powder* per day or equivalent vitamin-C rich foods.

Trace Minerals

⅛ – ½ teaspoon *Organic Kelp Powder* (for some people a smaller dose is better).

Fat-Soluble Vitamins A, D, and Activator X/"K2"

Taken with or before meals: (available at codliveroilshop.com)

¼ - ½ teaspoon *Blue Ice Royal Blend* 2-3 times per day (½ to 1 ½ teaspoons per day / 6-8 capsules)

or

½ to 1 teaspoon of real cod liver oil per day (make sure to take with 1 to 3 teaspoons of butter or ghee)

For synergistic effect add: ⅛ to ¼ teaspoon of *skate liver oil* (1-2 capsules)

Alternatives for those avoiding cod liver oil:

¼ to ¾ teaspoon daily of *skate liver oil* mixed with ½ to 2 teaspoons of ghee, or

⅓ to ¾ teaspoon daily of *X-Factor High Vitamin Butter Oil*

Gelatin and/or Broth

1-2 cups of homemade broth per day as a tea or with meals

or

½ to 1 tablespoon of gelatin reconstituted in water.

Liver from Any Animal

2+ ounces of fresh liver 2-4+ times per week and/or 1-3 teaspoons of *Dried Powdered Liver* 2-4 times per week (available at traditionalfoods.org).

Adequate Zinc

6 fresh oysters 2-4 times per week and/or 4-12 capsules of *Powdered Oysters* 2-4 times per week (available at traditionalfoods.org).

Alternative: If you are eating plenty of red meat like beef, lamb, and wild game, you are probably already getting adequate zinc. However these sources just do not have the magic that oysters have.

Good Salt – 1+ teaspoon per day of total dietary salt consumption.

Probiotic Foods – 1+ tablespoon of some type of fermented food of either vegetable or dairy origin, such as sauerkraut or fermented dairy like yogurt or kefir.

Spices – Make food flavorful to enhance digestion by using culinary spices in your dishes.

Optional yet Very Helpful

Bones and Cartilage: 2+ times per week consume some type of cooked or powdered bone. See chapter five for information about bone consumption from food.

Magnesium Baths or Topical Magnesium Oil: Apply 2+ times per week for magnesium supplementation. **This can be especially important if exclusively consuming bone calcium.**

Grass-fed Organ Meats: kidney, brain, tripe, "Rocky Mountain oysters," etc.

Fermented Dairy: include buttermilk, clabber, or whey for their healing benefits and calcium.

Essential Multi-Glandular: a blend of dried organs and glands such as thyroid, adrenals, pancreas, and gonads: to balance body chemistry and provide missing elements.

Organic Colostrum: to help rebuild the body and speed healing.

Fish Eggs: for trace elements and activator X/"K2."

Bone Marrow: or ½ teaspoon of freeze-dried bone marrow and cartilage powder to build teeth and bones.

Spirulina: rich in absorbable nutrients.

Coconut Oil: 1-3 teaspoons per day of coconut oil, for some people, can aid in overall body functioning, as well as enhance digestive function and liver health.[15]

Edible clay in small amounts: may provide trace minerals as well as absorb toxins in the body.

Many foods listed above are available at: traditionalfoods.org

Safer Carbohydrates (Choose Organic Where Possible)

White potatoes, sweet potatoes, yams, poi (taro root).

Organic sourdough bread from wheat, rye, spelt, etc. The bread should be made from flour that has most of the bran and germ removed. In other words, bread that is not 100 percent whole meal, but more precisely around 75-80 percent (with 20-25 percent of the fibrous grain portion by weight removed).

Beans that are smaller or easier to digest such as peas, lentils, black beans, and mung beans.

White rice, partially milled rice.

Nixtamalized (soaked in alkaline limewater and dehulled) organic corn tortillas.

Quinoa, amaranth, teff, soaked/soured buckwheat.

Vegetables: Most cooked organic vegetables are safe to consume in any amount.

Try a variety of different vegetables and see what works best for you.

Safe Fats:

The best and tastiest fats come from healthy animals.

Cultured butter or ghee from cultured butter is excellent.

Grass-fed beef tallow, pastured lard, pastured duck, chicken, goose, or turkey fat.

Organic coconut and palm oil, organic olive oil.

Strictly Moderate Consumption:

All nuts and nut products.

Entire (whole) grain products.

Exceptions: teff, amaranth, and quinoa are pseudo-cereals and not grains. Organic nixtamalized corn is from a whole grain, but the nixtamalization process neutralizes the toxins in corn. (Steer clear of genetically modified corn.)

And for some people with poor fat metabolism, reduce or avoid consumption of fatty foods and fatty cuts of meat like lamb and bacon.

Sweet ripe fruits.

Very sweet sweeteners—even natural ones like honey, maple syrup, and minimally processed natural sugar—need to be consumed with moderation.

Avoid Foods That Promote Inflammation or Calcium Loss

Some foods that are popular with health-conscious people should actually be avoided. Those who desire healthy teeth and gums would benefit from the following list of things to avoid:

No protein shakes

No energy bars or breakfast bars

No sweetened drinks

No beer, wine, or other alcohol (sorry)

No whole wheat bread

No packaged foods with added sweeteners, no matter how "natural"

No coffee

No caffeinated tea

No chocolate (very sorry)

No peanut butter

No white flour, store-bought, overly refined carbohydrate foods like pancakes, waffles, biscuits, pound cake, wheat / spelt / corn pasta, crackers.

Foods that Imbalance Body Chemistry and Promote Nutrient Depletion

This is a summary of foods to avoid that were discussed in greater detail in chapter six. Again, this list is to help you clarify which foods are going to deplete your body of nutrients and which foods are going to bring you back to life. The more disciplined you are in avoiding foods that cause or aggravate deficiency states in your body, the more successful you will be in healing gum disease, provided of course you continue to eat enough food. How you translate that guidance into action is totally your choice. I suggest that you give these guidelines your best attempt to follow and then judge how you feel.

Avoid sweets and foods sweetened with these items:

white sugar
cane sugar
evaporated cane juice
xylitol
agave nectar
jams
dried fruit
candy bars
"health food" bars
yacon syrup
erythritol
lo han
palm sugar
coconut sugar
stevia extract
glycerin
fructose
high fructose corn syrup
inulin
fructooligosaccharides (FOS)
brown rice syrup
malted barley
grain sweeteners
maltodextrin
sucrose
dextrose
sucralose
aspartame
saccharine

If you do not know what the sweetener is then avoid it.

Acceptable sweets in strict moderation:

unheated honey
organic maple syrup (grade B / very dark/strong taste preferred)
real cane sugar (Heavenly Organics™ or Rapunzel)
whole fruit including dates or fresh squeezed fruit juice

Avoid white flour or denatured grain products and strictly limit or avoid organically produced versions:

crackers
cookies
doughnuts
bagels
noodles
pies
breakfast cereals
granola
pasta
pizza
muffins
pastries
flour tortillas

Avoid bread even if it is organic unless it is sourdough from unbleached sifted (bran and germ free) grains, and nearly every packaged product that contains grains. Also avoid sprouted whole grain products and gluten-free foods made with brown rice.

Avoid whole grains that are not soured or sifted according to the guidelines in chapter six, including whole versions of: wheat, rye, kamut, spelt, or brown rice.

Acceptable grains: Sourdough bread made with unbleached flour (bran and germ removed), partially milled rice or white rice soaked overnight, nixtamalized organic corn tortillas, quinoa, amaranth, teff, and soaked/soured buckwheat.

Avoid raw nuts and nut butters including all raw nuts, as well as peanut butter, raw almond butter, and raw tahini. Too many nuts are harmful for people with significant gum recession.

Acceptable nuts and nut butters should be roasted or otherwise cooked. Low temperature dehydrated nuts and nut butters are acceptable in moderation.

Avoid partially hydrogenated oils such as margarine or other butter substitutes.

Avoid low quality vegetable oils such as vegetable, soybean, canola, corn, and safflower oils. Avoid potato chips, cottonseed oil, and any food not fried in a natural fat. Unfortunately most restaurants use these cheap vegetable oils, which makes their food unhealthy for regular consumption.

Acceptable fats are all natural, organic, and ideally from small producers. They include coconut oil, palm oil, olive oil, butter, lard, tallow, chicken, duck and goose fat.

Avoid pasteurized, homogenized, or grain-fed milk and ice cream. Also avoid low-fat conventional milk and powdered milk along with anything that contains it.

Acceptable Ice Cream: Make ice cream at home from fresh raw milk and cream and a natural sweetener. It is sooo good.

Avoid store-bought rice milk, soy milk, and nut milks like hemp and almond.

Acceptable milk alternatives: Make nut or seed milks at home—do not settle for store- bought sterilized versions.

Acceptable dairy products are raw and grass-fed from any type of ruminant and whole fat, not skimmed.

When you have only grocery store options for dairy products then organic unsweetened yogurt and butter are the best of the pasteurized dairy products. A good cheese selection will have some raw grass-fed cheeses. There are some acceptable pasteurized grass-fed cheeses from Australia, Ireland, and New Zealand that are reasonable in cost.

Avoid table salt: Many foods have commercial, refined salt added. Table salt seems highly irritating to the body perhaps because of its missing minerals, the additives, and substances used during the manufacture of it.[16]

Acceptable salts: Himalayan salt, *Celtic Sea Salt*®, and other sea salts are good to use.

Avoid conventional fast foods and junk foods. These foods are usually high in *trans* fats, food additive, and sugar.

Avoid stimulants: Do not drink coffee, sweetened drinks, or sports or energy drinks. Do not smoke cigarettes. Reduce or avoid chocolate.

Avoid alcohol: Alcohol is the enemy of calcium metabolism, and as such, it should be avoided—especially hard liquor. If you still choose to drink beer or wine, choose organic varieties as the grains or grapes can otherwise be heavily sprayed with pesticides.

Avoid unfermented soy in any form including isolated soy protein, tofu, soy/veggie burgers, soy "meat," and soy milk. Often gluten-free products contain hidden soy.

Acceptable soy products are traditionally fermented. Enjoy small amounts of unpasteurized soy sauce, miso, natto, and tempeh.

Caution with green powders: Most green powder supplements have sugar added and contain questionable ingredients. There are a few exceptions to this rule, which would be 100 percent food-based dried powders with no sweeteners added.

Avoid factory-farmed meat, fish, and eggs. These offer inferior quality proteins, support the unhealthy treatment of animals and regular consumption may cause or contribute to cancer.[17]

Acceptable animal proteins are grass-fed or wild. These offer superior quality and bolster health and also support a healthy ecosystem.

Avoid too much fruit. Even though fruit is natural, people often eat too much. Be very careful with sweet fruits like oranges, bananas, grapes, peaches, cherries, blueberries, and pineapple. This caution also includes excess consumption of unripe fruit because they are high in salicylates and in general upset digestion.

Avoid prescription drugs, over-the-counter drugs, and vaccines. These alter your glandular balance and many can be causative factors in gum disease. Vaccines can contain substances very toxic to the body. Prescription drugs often treat symptoms and not the core problem, and as a result have unwanted side effects.

Avoid food additives like MSG. In addition many mass-produced commercially cured and processed meats contain preservatives that are irritating to the body.

Avoid commercially processed foods such as TV dinners and packaged sauce mixes.

Avoid synthetic vitamins and any foods containing them. I believe the whole food approach is a more effective way to nourish our bodies.

Body Chemistry Balancing Diet to Restore Gum Health

Gluten-Free and Mostly Dairy-Free/Paleo Style

This dairy-free and grain-free diet is meant to help balance your body chemistry and is based on the work of dentist Melvin Page.[18,19] This plan should help improve your health by balancing body chemistry, which can positively affect the gum health. The first sign that it is working is some temporary detoxification symptoms like headaches, chills, and fatigue. (These should not last more than a few days.) Try this plan for one to four weeks if you feel like your body needs a reset. After the initial period, you can expand to the general dietary plan if you like.

This diet consists of a protein element, a moderate amount of fat, and plenty of vegetables with every meal. Make sure to eat plenty of calories when implementing this plan and do not deprive yourself of what you need.

Body Chemistry Balancing Diet Notes:

- ☐ This is not meant to be a high protein and low fat diet; if you need to increase your protein intake, make sure you increase your fat intake by just as much or more. Otherwise, consuming too much protein without the balancing fat can become toxic.
- ☐ If you need to increase your calorie intake, consider starchy foods like winter squashes and sweet potatoes.
- ☐ Not all people need to avoid dairy completely for this dietary reset. Ghee should work well for people who are dairy sensitive.
- ☐ If you absolutely must avoid dairy completely, then I would recommend good beef or bison tallow, preferably from rendered kidney fat.

Body Chemistry Balancing Food Plan

6+ ounces of protein per day from healthy animal sources such as pastured chicken, turkey, pork, beef, and/or from wild fish such as tuna, salmon, and sardines.

Healthy Fat: ½ - 3 tablespoons of grass-fed butter or ghee, cultured preferred.

Vegetables: Plenty of vegetables of any sort to go with your protein. The following list is just a sampling as any vegetable you feel drawn to you can include in your diet: beet greens, kale, lettuce, collard greens, cucumber, chard, celery, cauliflower, broccoli, bok choy, salad greens, zucchini, and string beans.

Starches: Starches are not required, but they will help you get plenty of calories and feel full. Safe starches for body chemistry balancing are sweet potatoes; yams; taro root; acorn, butternut, summer, and winter squashes; pumpkin; carrots; beets; turnips; and rutabagas.

Gelatin, and/or Broth

1-2 cups of homemade broth per day as a tea or with meals

or

½ to 1 tablespoon of gelatin reconstituted in water.

Liver from any Animal Source: 2+ ounces of fresh liver 2-4+ times per week and/or 1-3 teaspoons of *Dried Powdered Liver* 2-4 times per week (available at traditionalfoods.org).

Adequate Zinc: 6 fresh oysters 2-4 times per week and/or 4-12 capsules of *Powdered Oysters* 2-4 times per week (available at traditionalfoods.org).

Probiotic Foods: 1+ tablespoon of some type of fermented vegetable such as sauerkraut.

Good Salt: 1+ teaspoon per day of total dietary salt consumption.

Supplements - Most people should take these 4-6 days per week and not every day to allow the body to recalibrate.

Calcium: 1½-3 teaspoons *Bone Marrow & Cartilage* (600mg – 1,200mg) (or for those who can do dairy, fermented liquid dairy products like kefir or yogurt).

Trace Minerals: ⅛–½ teaspoon *Organic Kelp Powder* (for some people a smaller dose is better).

Vitamin C: ¼–2 teaspoons of *High Vitamin C powder* per day or equivalent vitamin C-rich foods.

Fat-Soluble Vitamins A, D, and Activator X/"K2"

(See the **general dietary guidelines** earlier in this chapter. These vitamins are essential; do not skip them.)

Optional: Some people will benefit by eating 4-6 smaller meals per day instead of two or three larger ones.

Foods to Avoid for the Body Chemistry Diet Plan In addition to avoiding the foods listed in the **general dietary plan,** this plan excludes nuts, seeds, beans, fruits, grains, corn, pseudo-cereals, regular potatoes, and cheese.

For the longer term, this body chemistry diet plan is fairly restrictive and may be limiting some foods that your body craves. In the long run, you can modify this diet how you like by combining it with principles from the general diet plan to accommodate other dietary preferences such as paleo, grain-free, dairy-free, and gluten-free. The key is to use your best judgment and if something continually does not feel good or does not work for you, change course and get additional support. Remember, these guidelines are not meant to cause food deprivation or orthorexia, an unhealthy obsession with eating healthy.

Extreme / Therapeutic Gum Disease Reversing Diet

Raw primal diets are based on the late and outside-the-box nutritionist Aajonus Vonderplanitz. His dietary guide is *The Recipe for Living without Disease.* Some people following such a diet experience excellent health and healing over time, even with "hopeless" cases for whom no other treatment has worked. The highlight and basic concept is that uncooked animal fats and proteins are easiest to digest. Of course, use these guidelines at your own responsibility and adapt them to work for your body. This is not a "one size fits all" approach and these guidelines may need modification if you choose to follow a diet like this.

2–4 cups of vegetable juice daily between meals (see green juice recipe in chapter seven)
8+ ounces raw organic meat, chicken, or wild fish per day [organic often means grain-fed]
6 raw oysters per day
4 ounces of raw grass-fed cheese
2-4 ounces raw grass-fed butter per day
4-8 raw pastured eggs per day
4-8 cups raw grass-fed milk, yogurt, or kefir per day*
1 tablespoon raw grass-fed bone marrow
1-2 ounces of raw grass-fed liver
⅛–½ teaspoon organic kelp powder

Fat-soluble vitamins

½-1¼ Green Pasture Cod Liver Oil / Butter Oil Mix (Blue Ice Royal Blend)
¼-½ teaspoon Skate Liver Oil

Optional Supplements

1 teaspoon organic colostrum
Other raw organs and glands
1 teaspoon *Essential Multi-Glandular* (if not consuming raw organs and glands)
½-1 teaspoon *Bone, Marrow, and Cartilage* (if not consuming bone marrow)

*lesser amounts of raw cheese can be used to replace the milk.

This raw diet can also be modified into a semi-raw diet by cooking or searing the animal foods, creating a diet that is low in dietary fiber with easy-to-absorb milk, meat, fat, and vegetable juice.

Simple Cure Gum Disease Program

If you find the advice in this book too much or too hard to follow, then try to break the program down into one or two dietary concepts that most appeal to you. Here is a simple program to help you get started in which you can improve your nutrition but without having to make any significant changes.

Simple Diet and Health Plan

1. Consume grass-fed butter as your main source of fat.
2. Follow the calcium suggestions from the general diet plan to ensure adequate calcium intake.
3. Take kelp powder daily or sprinkle kelp powder on many foods.
4. Avoid refined / very sweet sweeteners.
5. Exercise or engage in movement such as walking at least two to four times per week.

Add-ons (Other Important Ideas)

1. Cod liver oil / butter oil mix (*Blue Ice Royal Blend*) (codliveroilshop.com).
2. Avoid gluten.
3. Consume soup made with bones.

4. Take an *Essential Multi-Glandular* supplement to help balance body chemistry (traditionalfoods.org).
5. Consume *High Vitamin C powder* (traditionalfoods.org).

Precautions for High Fat, High Protein, Grain-Rich Diet That Avoids Dairy and/or Seafood with Respect to Gum Disease

Dentist George Heard (author of *Man vs. Toothache*) linked gum disease to a diet heavy in meat, gravy, bread, and potatoes.[20] Too much meat and animal fat consumed for a long time without enough calcium and trace minerals can cause the bone structure to waste away.[21] One reason this occurs is because grains and animal flesh are very high in phosphorus. Because a diet high in phosphorous and low in calcium leads to gum disease, proteins and grains need to be balanced with plenty of calcium and trace minerals. Likewise, a high fat diet requires minerals in our body for metabolism, as much as the minerals need the fat to be utilized correctly and efficiently by the body. If you eat a high fat diet, balance it with mineral-dense foods like seaweed and dairy products, or a bone-based calcium supplement.

Be Patient with Getting Results from Dietary Changes: Time Is Essential

For many of us, our bodies have endured years if not decades of a nutrient-deficient diet. The toll this has taken on our bodies has resulted in poor overall health and specifically mineral depletion in our jaws and supporting tissues, resulting in inflammation and tissue destruction known as gum disease. Because of the long, slow process for disease to form, it may take an equal amount of time to see satisfying results and to repair the damage done. Give yourself at least two months to see some results (of course they can happen much faster!), and at least six months and up to a year or longer to see more definitive and permanent changes. As you are following a healthy diet, you should be feeling better and better and have a sense of well being more and more. If you do not continue to feel better and instead start feeling worse, then seek additional support, as something is going awry. If you are feeling better but are not seeing the results you had hoped for, then it is time to be patient and to find additional ways to evaluate if your health goal is being satisfied.

Common Diet Mistakes That Produce Less Ideal Results

Everyone is unique and faces different challenges. Here are some things to watch out for if you are not experiencing the degree of gum healing you may have expected:

Poor food quality: Absolutely avoid packaged foods, even foods labeled organic, as they may not truly nourish you. If you are a great fan of dairy products, be aware that grain-fed dairy products, even if they are raw, can cause imbalances. Get the best and freshest food you are able to find.

Skipping fat-soluble vitamins: Fat-soluble vitamins are of utmost importance in nourishing strong alveolar bones and supporting tissues, especially vitamin D. If you skip this step, restoring gum health can be difficult to achieve.

Too much sweet food: A sweet is a sweet. If you have gum disease, you must limit your sweets. Your gums are worth it. Natural sweets are safer than highly refined ones, but there is a point at which you may suffer consequences.

Lack of minerals: Bone broth aids in nutrient absorption and is rich in minerals. Seaweed, fish, and shellfish are very rich in minerals. Calcium is critical for those suffering from gum disease.

Poor food absorption: Perhaps you are not digesting your food well. Focus on adding fermented foods, bone broth, kefir, and raw eggs, to aid in digestion. Perhaps you need to reconsider a deeper cleanse or detoxification as discussed in chapter seven. Many times chronically poor digestion can be the result of heavy metal poisoning, particularly from mercury, or scar tissue that resulted from large doses of antibiotics. You may need some of digestive aids recommended in chapter seven.

Eating Good Food Now that you know the outline of what to eat and what to avoid, you have the rewarding challenge of converting these ideas into meals and menus. At **curegumdisease.com/food** you will find a list of suggested cookbooks and online resources you can use to find recipes that in general complement the dietary advice in this book. Listed below are also some grain-free meal ideas to get you started. These do not necessarily represent an ideal diet, but are a good start for a balanced diet.

Meal Ideas: These can be served at any meal of the day—breakfast, lunch, or dinner. Making lunch the biggest meal of the day may work well for some readers.

Scrambled eggs, milk, fresh salad
Soft-boiled eggs
Fish fried or steamed with vegetables and potatoes, yams, or sweet potatoes
Potatoes, steamed beef, chicken, or fish, carrots, stewed fruit
Lamb or mutton stew made with soup bones and potatoes, with cooked fruit and milk
Chicken soup with vegetables
Fish head soup
Clam, mussel, or oyster chowder
Sushi, miso soup made with fish broth and seaweed
Ceviche with crispy corn tortillas
Seafood stew (cioppino) with fish stock, fish, squid, mussels, and clams; toasted sourdough bread, rice or potatoes
Meat loaf made with 25 percent ground organ meats, cooked in beef stock Butternut squash soup made with chicken broth
Shrimp, chicken, or lamb kabobs with liver, heart and/or kidney, grilled with assorted vegetables (peppers, zucchini, mushrooms) tossed in oil, sea salt, pepper, and sides of broth and corn on the cob
Steak tartare with raw ground beef
Potato cakes or fish cakes
Fish and potatoes
Lentil or celery soup made with milk and chopped chicken or beef
Cheese, served in various ways, with meats and pickled vegetables
Beef, turkey, or chicken meatballs in beef broth, marinara sauce with vegetables topped with cheese. Or meat balls with spaghetti squash
Liver with caramelized onions
Roasted bone marrow on sourdough bread

Snacks should include both some protein and some fat, such as:

Milk, yogurt, cheese, kefir, beef jerky (with some butter or beef fat)

Dairy Tips:

If you are consuming large amounts of fluid milk or yogurt, try consuming them away from meals that contain other animal protein, as it may make it easier to digest.

In the Aruyvedic tradition, raw fresh milk is brought to a gentle boil for one to five minutes and mixed with spices like turmeric, ginger, and cardamom to create a milk tea. Usually a touch of sweetener is then added. In the same tradition, yogurt can be mixed with water and spices to form a digestive aid called a Lassi. For specific instructions, visit curegumdisease.com/milk

If you "need" to have a sweet, have it in the middle of the day so that there is time for your blood sugar to stabilize rather than after dinner when it could affect your sleep.

Examples of healthier sweets:

(Hint: In general use less sweetener than is suggested in recipes.)

Fresh fruit salad with egg custard or cream
Baked apple, center filled with maple syrup with ice cream
Homemade ice-cream with raw milk / cream and using a modest amount of sweetener like honey or maple syrup
Rice pudding made with white rice
Homemade Jello with good gelatin
Homemade cheesecake

After reading through this entire book and learning step-by-step how this dietary advice came about, I hope that you have a reasonable grasp on what causes gum disease, and how to make real and lasting changes in your life. Next, let's take a look at the different treatment options available at your dentist and periodontist so you can create an integrative treatment plan for healing gum disease naturally.

9 Dentistry and Gum Disease

Dentists are surgeons. D.D.S. stands for Doctor of Dental Surgery. Dentists are trained to do surgery on your mouth to repair a problem. Surgery comes at substantial price: it is often painful, it can result in permanent tissue changes, it often exposes you to toxic substances, and it can be expensive. If this pain results in healing, then it is a worthy sacrifice. *But all too often* the physical pain, the financial pain, and the emotional pain are not only ineffective in the long run, but completely unnecessary.

Dental Trauma and Abuse

Any treatment done to our bodies that is unnecessary is a form of physical abuse and invasion. Our mouths, being a sensitive orifice in our body, are a center of nourishment and pleasure. When we allow someone to do things to our mouth, our consent is only based on the belief that this type of touch, or possible medical procedure, will significantly benefit our health. When we agree to a dental treatment, it means we have chosen to pay a certain price in terms of pain and in terms of allowing a professional to manipulate, investigate, and potentially cut a part of our body. When this treatment is done from a place of fear, whereby we may have felt manipulated, not only does it not serve us, it becomes traumatic.

Sometimes children are subjected to medical or dental treatments that they do not understand. Not only do they not understand what the medical intervention is, they often do not have a choice in the matter. Choice is essential in understanding what creates a traumatic response in the body. When we feel we choose something, then we can go along with the treatment and accept the resulting pain. But when we feel something is imposed upon us, we resist and we fight against the experience. And each consequence of the action we feel we did not choose can become a great source of pain in our lives.

I myself am a "victim" for lack of a better word, of dental abuse. Many people I have communicated with have shared how they've felt mistreated by their dentist. It can leave one feeling inwardly incomplete, and often times quite angry. For me, it was unnecessary and very aggressive orthodontics when I was a child. So I understand keenly the experience of being compelled to do something that does not feel right, and then feeling shame and defeat when left with the possibility of permanent and debilitating changes having been done to one's body.

Therefore, in order to cast a protective shield around patients who approach this profession that has too often crossed boundaries with the treatments performed, I am generally supportive of the most sensitive and least invasive treatment approach. I favor dental treatments, which do not involve cutting, poisoning, and destroying, and prefer treatments that feel healing, revitalizing, and renewing. Not only do I prefer a treatment that feels life affirming, I also seek the experience of being received and held compassionately by a dentist who is radiating positive and caring energy because he or she is truly aligned with helping, and supporting . . . and not hurting.

Because the potential for trauma and abuse in a dental office is high, many people become terrified when thinking of visiting a dentist or about a particular treatment approach. Furthermore, confusion is created when they have treatments pushed at them that are injurious and done under the guise of routine care. When a treatment feels forced, the person loses their own volition or choice in the matter, and it can become traumatic, or at least feel abusive to people who experience this kind of treatment. One example is dental X-rays. In certain situations, a dental X-ray or CT scan could help to clarify a specific problem and treatment approach. But dental X-rays significantly increase the risk of both thyroid cancer[1] and brain cancer.[2] Ironically, dental X-rays are irradiating the most important glands for calcium metabolism, the thyroid and the pituitary. Despite this very real concern, for legal reasons and profit, dental X-rays are done more often than necessary. When a treatment is done that is not necessary, it hurts the body.

If you have experienced dental trauma or abuse in the past from an unnecessary or overly invasive treatment, there are a few things you can do to help. First, just notice or acknowledge what feelings you have in relation to the procedure done, even if it is uncomfortable. Give yourself space to have whatever feelings you have. If that is not enough, I think cranial-sacral treatment is the best modality to unwind physical stress in the body. Look for a practitioner who does work in the mouth; for example, some practitioners can release stuck TMJ joints, or rotated teeth, by doing intra-oral treatments.

Gum Disease Is a Nutrient Problem, so Why Operate?

Most periodontists and dentists proceed on the false theory that oral disease can be cured by the removal of bacterial plaque, but as was discussed in chapters one and three, the removal of bacterial plaque rarely if ever results in a cure for gum disease. Dentists think that gum disease is incurable because their treatments do not cure it, and so most of them have resigned themselves to merely treat the symptoms of gum disease. Because they often cannot facilitate a cure, they erroneously conclude that no cure exists. If a cure existed, then they would have no justification or reasons for prescribing many of the treatments for gum disease.

Modern dentists need to become bold enough to look at the rest of the body and not just the mouth. They could then see that surgical treatments should be a last resort, and not the first line of treatment for periodontitis. Periodontal treatments are founded upon a false belief system that focuses on bacteria as the cause of gum disease, which ignores the latest evidence that shows that the health of the individual is what creates immunity to gum disease. If the premise behind the treatment paradigm is flawed, then a question to ponder is whether the prescribed treatments for gum disease will be effective or even necessary?

Finding a Good Dentist or the Right Treatment

Finding a good dentist and knowing what treatments you need and want is often a challenging and frustrating experience for people. I believe that when you see the bigger picture, as I am about to describe, it will help explain why there is often confusion about finding a good dentist and finding a treatment protocol that actually helps.

Some dental heroes still do exist. They have long ago abandoned obsolete belief systems and have seen the horror of unnecessary and toxic dental work. Usually they are quietly doing good dental work and helping patients find their way back to health by undoing and redoing the often unnecessary and poorly done dental work of other dentists. Your job as a patient seeking excellent treatment and care is to align yourself and locate such a dentist for such support. But I will warn you, for some people it is not only difficult, but impossible to find a positive dentist in their area, so if you need more support, you will not only need to look deeply and thoroughly, but also look far away. For example, when I got my mercury fillings removed, I interviewed dentists on the phone and then flew to another state. It was worth it to find a dentist that was aligned with performing the mercury removal in a way that I felt would best support my health. As a result of my diligence and extra effort, there was no pain involved in the procedure and I felt quite elated and relieved on my way home.

When seeking a good dentist or periodontist, look for someone who is willing to take the time to explain to you what the dental or periodontal treatment they recommend entails. A good dentist will not try to push you, scare you, or coerce you into submitting to a treatment. Fear is an effective motivator to force a patient to submit, but it is not informed consent, nor is it ethical to use. Trauma and abuse happens in dentistry when the patient is not ready or willing to receive the treatment, and so the treatment is forced upon the patient.

A good dentist or periodontist wants to get to know who you are as a person. If they take the effort to see you as a person, then the odds of them pushing an unnecessary treatment on you decrease significantly. Performing good dentistry is an art, and good dental work takes not only an artistic hand, but a good mind to accurately diagnose the patient and give them a treatment that supports their healing process. When you feel unsure or unclear about a prescribed treatment, my suggestion is to get more information. Often clarifying and understanding the details of the recommended procedure will make it very obvious if the treatment is right for you or not. Do not consent to treatments based upon blind faith on authorities, and hope that is right for you. Instead, become a periodontal detective in search of the best treatment for you.

Things to Consider When Choosing a Dental or Periodontal Procedure

- ☐ Ask for before and after case studies with pictures and/or X-rays.
- ☐ Talk to patients who have undergone the same treatment that you are considering from the same dentist.
- ☐ Ask for studies proving the efficacy of the treatment recommended.
- ☐ Ask for a less invasive treatment first to see if your problem will be corrected with the simpler and less costly procedure.

A Second Opinion

If you feel unsure about the treatment or recommendation of your dentist, consider getting another opinion from a different dentist. Different dentists may have different treatment philosophies and/or techniques. Of course if you happen to be lucky and find a good dentist whom you trust and who uses minimally invasive dentistry, then getting another opinion could lead you astray. In the end, do what is necessary to give yourself the effort you deserve. It can be more work, but if it leads you to getting a better treatment, it will be worth it.

The Patient's Dilemma about Gum Disease Treatment

There often seems to be so much pain, turmoil, fear, and frustration when it comes to choosing a periodontal or dental treatment. Because of this, by far, the most common question I am asked is whether someone needs or can avoid a certain treatment prescribed by their dentist. (Please note: I neither prescribe treatments nor recommend avoiding dentists entirely, not only for legal reasons, but because I do not have or want to take the authority to know what is right for someone else to do with their body. It is each person's individual choice.) An example of this dilemma is that, today, as I am writing this, I just talked with someone because their dentist recently told them the bad news—that their gum disease is incurable, and that the only treatment for them is gum surgery. Let's look at some reasons why this happens to many people.

The reason there is so much confusion and frustration for patients is often because dentists only make money when they perform a service or treatment. This leads to a common occurrence of overtreatment. Investigative journalist William Ecenbarger visited fifty random dental offices across the country in 1997 for their treatment recommendations for a dental problem. Twenty out of the fifty offices (40 percent) recommended significantly more dental work than two expert dentists who carefully reviewed his case said he actually needed. In the most extreme case of the twenty overzealous treatment programs, one dentist in New York City recommended twenty-one unnecessary crowns at the cost of $29,850 for Mr. Ecenbarger. Three out of fifty dentists (6 percent) said he had no problems at all, and twelve out of fifty dentists (24 percent) agreed with the expert findings. Much to the chagrin of the dental profession, he published the results of his research in a Readers Digest article titled, "How Dentists Rip Us Off."[3]

Many dentists have put their licenses on the line to expose this overtreatment and fraud that is rampant in the dental industry. Here are a few examples: Dentist Robert Nara wrote *Money by the Mouthful*, dentist Marvin Schissel wrote *Dentistry and Its Victims*, Dentist Hal Huggins wrote *It's All in Your Head*, and Dr. Graeme Munro-Hall wrote *Toxic Dentistry Exposed.*

As I continue to share about the common hazards in the dental field, consider taking a moment to notice how this affects you. Do you agree with me? Does this make you feel angry? Or sad? Just notice how you inwardly respond and allow whatever response there is to be present. When I started researching dental health ten years ago, I came from a perspective of innocence. I was not looking for problems; I was looking for solutions. I have learned from other dentists, reading, and other people's experiences that dentistry in general no longer offers the best for its patients.

And I need to share what I know, so that it can inspire dialogue and change in dentistry and periodontology where innovations are truly needed and beneficial.

I became clear about the all too common fraud and abuse in the dental profession after a dentist with a very extensive résumé contacted me. While I cannot say their name, this dentist wanted me to be absolutely clear about one thing: a large majority of dentists are not to be trusted. This dentist did not just tell me this; they follow this principal with their actions. When this dentist's friend went in for a dental checkup, the dentist personally called the office while I was on the other phone line, to let them know that the patient was friends with the powerful dentist, so as to protect the patient from unnecessary treatment.

Besides medical doctors, the dental profession has the highest suicide rate[4], and alcoholism is a common problem. The cause could be mercury poisoning, which many dentists suffer from, from placing and removing mercury fillings without adequate protective gear. It could also be from what happens to the individual's soul when they perform treatments to make money which are not helping people. It could also be from how in the past dental school education was often emotionally abusive to students. If dentists are not treated with respect as students, then they won't likely treat their staff, their patients, or even themselves with respect either.

Just like with politics, part of the root of the problem in the dental field is money. Placing the profit motive above all else is a dire error when it comes to medical and dental care. Dentists are often trained by sales people to sell more treatments and to prescribe add-ons such as X-rays, much like what often happens when you go to a car dealership for an oil change. This is done primarily for the purpose of increasing their income by selling more services and not because it supports the overall health and well-being of the patient.

Even with a dentist trying to do their best, the treatment model for periodontal disease is often flawed. Dentists have many tools and treatment techniques that they want to use. They want to use what they have learned to help people. But often times, the patient is made to fit into a treatment that is not right for them, because the dentist has a limited set of tools that they can offer. And if the patient does not fit into what is available, there is no money to be made. No matter how excellent the surgeon or the dental technology, it is only of benefit to you if you actually need the treatment. The best treatment modalities and procedures are not the status quo in the field of dentistry. For example, consider mercury fillings, which has been a foundational treatment for tooth decay. Mercury is more toxic than plutonium, and even though this is an undisputed fact, dentists are still implanting it in people's heads! Not only does mercury poison and pollute the body, dentists flush the mercury-rich water down the drain, polluting the environment.

Despite these hurdles, not all dentists are flawed. You do not necessarily need to flee the country for dental work, although for some it might be a good idea. Rather, it means that I do not recommend that you give your trust to a dentist lightly or haphazardly. The few, hard to find "gem" dentists, periodontists, or hygienists will show you through their thoughts, actions, feelings, and treatments that they genuinely care for you and your health more than they care about making money. If the person you are working with does not care about you and you feel that you are simply an object to add to the dentist's bank account, then I advise you to leave immediately and do not return. You can go to curegumdisease.com/dentist which will direct you to lists of dentists who are more likely to, but not necessarily going to, offer holistic and supportive treatments.

Beyond the systemic issues of dentistry from the conventional perspective, the dental field ignores nutritional research which, as you now know, is essential for better treatment outcomes, less invasive treatment models, and for preventing and healing gum disease naturally.

The Dentist's Dilemma

A typical dentist goes to school for four years to obtain a bachelor's degree, and then goes for an additional four years of education in dental school to become a dentist. To become a specialist, two or more additional years of postgraduate work are required. After this extensive education, the *average* dental school graduate in the U.S. is $241,000 in debt by the time they finish dental school.[5] This figure does not include the cost of starting a practice. In some countries such as Switzerland and Germany, dentists do not graduate with debt because of government subsidized education. Therefore, in other places in the world, dentistry can be better than in the U.S. because the incentive structure and belief systems are different.

The youthful dental student would not usually consider that university dental education could possibly be defective. Why would one expect that this prestigious and expensive education would teach anything but the best science and the whole truth? But the education is completely biased toward solely promoting a system of dental surgery and excluding all other thought or alternative knowledge. Dental students are not taught about the discoveries of the famous dentists who preceded them and tackled challenging dental problems at their very core, like Price, Page, and Hawkins. The very real and important critiques and studies done on the dental field are not incorporated into the teaching; for example, toxic filling materials are still used as if it does not matter what type of material is implanted into people's teeth. And the newly minted dentists are eager to begin their practices, apply what they have learned, and they completely expect to make a handy profit.

Just as the dentist has been trained to be a skilled technician in the repair of teeth and gums, he or she has patients lining up with their dental dilemmas. According to the standard medical model, there is no need for patients to do that much to take care of themselves or to change anything in their behavior, because for a price, dentists will fix whatever problem they have. The dentists' dilemma is that they have bills to pay, pressure to perform, and an expectation that they are the demigods of the mouth. They are here to triumph over evil bacteria and rescue the helpless patients who have come to them for tooth and gum salvation. So dentists dutifully do what they were taught to do in dental school.

In general, dentists are skeptical about how nutrition relates to gum disease and tooth decay, because how could it be possible that if nutrition was so important, that government health departments, insurance companies, dental schools, dental health boards, and dental associations would not know or inform about this information? The curative power of nutrition, while interesting and possibly even useful, is discounted in favor of drilling, scraping, cutting, and implanting. The struggle of the dentist is that the truth about what really causes tooth decay and gum disease is profoundly at odds with what he or she has been taught and practiced. To consider that the entire paradigm of dental care is built upon false foundations and misconceptions is all too painful, too shameful, and too horrifying to accept.

Your Feelings Matter; Listen to Them

Harness the intelligence of your feelings as well as the sensations in your body to your advantage by noticing how you feel in response to your dentist. When you hear or think of a specific dental treatment, acknowledge the felt sense response. This feeling response can be a useful tool in helping you decide what treatment to undertake. For example, notice if you feel relieved and reassured after your initial dental consultation, or discouraged and daunted. Before accepting any treatment, ask yourself, "Is this right for me?" After all, it is your mouth and your body. You have the right to choose or refuse treatments. Informed consent means that the choice is always yours!

Understanding the Conventional System

In the field of periodontology, most practitioners have been trained to perform the same procedures and it is rare to find those who innovate from creativity and inspiration in seeking new ways to provide effective treatments. Even with this high degree of similarity of perspective, there are significant disagreements in the field as to when and which treatments are best to perform. As a result, this section aims to give as much evidence and clarity as possible regarding treatment options, while leaving the final treatment decision up to you. In addition, because there is so much disagreement on certain topics, some of the discussion of treatment options may not feel as complete as could be ideal. So, this is meant to be an overview to help inspire you in the right direction, but further investigation may be required on your end.

Periodontal Probing

Periodontal probing is not usually a pleasant procedure, and little has changed in the past hundred years in terms of the technique.[6] A small, thin, usually metallic probe is slid between the teeth and gum line. Measurements, in millimeters, are taken as to how deep the periodontal pocket is. For perspective, one inch is 25.4 millimeters (mm) and there are 10 mm in 1 centimeter. The purpose of probing is not only to see how deep the pockets are, but also to measure how far the gum line (gingival margin) has receded from its ideal position. The ideal position of the gums is just slightly elevated above the cemento-enamel junction, the meeting place of the cementum of the tooth and the enamelized crown of the tooth. Probing can induce bleeding, which happens when already inflamed and sensitive tissue

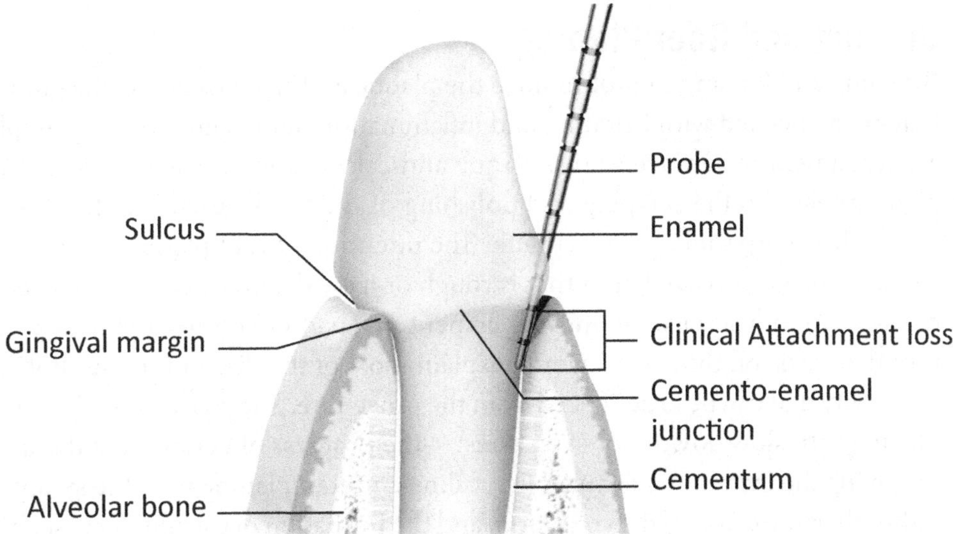

is prodded. If the sites probed do not bleed, it generally means that inflammation is minimal.

Accurate dental probing aims to document clinical attachment level (CAL) and probing depth (PD) to measure the progression of gum disease.

Clinical attachment level (CAL) refers to how far the gum has detached from its original position. This measures not only how deep the gum pocket is, but also how deep the gum pocket is in relation to the original height of the gum tissue.

Probing depth (PD) simply measures how deep the pocket is relative to the height of the gingival margin (gum line). If the gum line is receded, the probing depth could be small, but there could still be significant gum recession. The CAL measurement represents how far the gum has receded from its original position.

What Is the Difference between a Periodontist and a Dentist?

Periodontists are dentists who specialize in the prevention, diagnosis, and treatment of periodontal disease, and in the placement of dental implants.[7] Most general dentists attempt to manage periodontal disease in their offices with scaling and root planing. Periodontists generally take patients with the most challenging or severe cases related to gum recession. They furthermore do gum implants and other gum surgeries.

Scaling and Root Planing

Brushing and flossing cannot remove the plaque and calculus below the gum line that are associated with irritation and inflammation of the gums. Scaling employs an instrument to remove stains, plaque and calculus below the gum line.[8] Root planing refers to the scraping and polishing of the tooth surface under the gum line with a sharp tool called a curette. The intention of root planing is to remove cementum and surface dentin that is rough or has calculus or bacteria in order to create a smooth surface.[9] Removing cementum (part of your tooth) with a sharp tool that peels off thin layers would explain most of the discomfort and hot/cold sensitivity that can be experienced from the procedure. The goal of scaling and root planing is to slow down—or even arrest—the progress of periodontal disease by removing the irritant. Unfortunately, scaling and root planing treat the symptoms rather than the cause of the condition, and the formation of calculus almost always continues after the treatment.[10] Therefore, people with periodontal disease end up being frequent repeat candidates for this procedure.

Note: As I discuss the various dental procedures, keep in mind that the perspective I am coming from is that I am not "recommending" them, but trying to inform you about them so you can clearly understand the possible benefits or detriments.

The Many Types of Scaling and Root Planing

As it turns out, the aggressive procedure of removing the cementum of the tooth as done in traditional root planing to create a smooth and glassy tooth root surface is not necessary to reduce the inflammation caused by periodontal disease.[11] It should be common sense to know that removing tooth structure, as the root planing procedure is intended to do, will traumatize the periodontium.[12] A 2004 study showed that using curettes for scaling and root planing (SRP) causes on average 0.76 mm (millimeters) of attachment loss due to trauma from the procedure.[13]

A new scaling and root planing (SRP) methodology that preserves the cementum has been developed called *periodontal debridement*. Most dentists are not familiar with the specific meaning of the term *debridement*, because the term has not been embraced by the American Dental Association. The newer, less invasive SRP modality focuses on primarily using ultrasonic instruments to clean plaque and calculus while significantly reducing or eliminating the usual carving away and smoothing of the tooth root (root planing). The new method asserts that endotoxins do not penetrate the cementum, and so the removal of cementum is not necessary. Discomfort after scaling and root planing will be significantly reduced when the cementum is left intact.

Clearly the least invasive form of SRP is better for you as it preserves tooth structure. The only way you are going to know what method your hygienist, dentist, or periodontist uses is to ask. Before you make any appointment, discover if they primarily use ultrasonic tools, if they remove any cementum, if they use a curette, and if their focus is on preserving tooth structure. If you do not get a clear answer or promise from the dental office that they use this less invasive cleaning procedure, then move on and find a place that will provide you with root cleaning that preserves your periodontium.

More about Scaling and Root Planing

Scaling and root planing (SRP) is considered the indispensible, most effective standard of care for the in-office treatment of gum disease that your dentist or periodontist can provide. Therefore it is the standard phase 1 in-office treatment for patients with gum disease. The effectiveness of the SRP method should be evaluated over a period of three to six months before moving to more invasive phase 2 surgical procedures.[14]

Scaling and root planning should only be performed on teeth with a 4mm or deeper pocket depth. Root scaling teeth with less than 4mm (1-3mm) pocket depth (as measured from the depth of the cemento-enamel junction) will cause damage to the tooth root.[15] Keep in mind that SRP without any other intervention cannot put gum disease into permanent remission, because gum disease is caused by biochemistry imbalances (host response), and not from an absence of tooth cleaning or gum surgery.

Patients should be charged per tooth rather than per quadrant unless all of the teeth in the quadrant are affected. If the pocket depth has not significantly decreased three months after a scaling and root planing procedure, many conventional dentists consider the patient a candidate for more extensive, expensive, and invasive surgery. However if most of the pockets are less than 6mm, a more appropriate course of action would be more cleaning and scaling over the course of the next year.[16] The need for periodontal surgery should be approached cautiously and conservatively, but far too often surgery is done to benefit the surgeon's pocket book rather than meeting the patient's needs.[17] Periodontal disease is usually a slow progressing disease and there is generally no need to rush into surgery due to the expected periods of remission.[18] Even the American Academy of Periodontology agrees that scaling and root planing is sufficient treatment for gum disease and that "many patients do not require any further active treatment, including surgical therapy."[19]

The Effectiveness of Scaling and Root Planing

On average, pocket reduction from scaling and root planing of deep pockets is 1.3-2.2mm (millimeters) and bleeding of the unhealthy pockets is reduced by 57 percent. However, on shallow pockets of 1-4 mm, SRP causes an average 0.3mm attachment **loss.**[20] Clearly, scaling and root planing is *not* a good treatment paradigm for shallow gum pockets.

With deeper pockets of 4-7mm, the average is 0.55mm of attachment gain from SRP, and for pockets greater than 6mm, an average gain of 1.19mm.[21] However, even with these apparent gains, gingival recession often continues or recurs.[22] In others words, it is possible to have both gingival recession and attachment gain from the same procedure. This is when the gum pocket shrinks, and the gum line still recedes. This leads me to make three suggestions for those who opt for scaling and root planing procedures:

1. Eat a good diet beforehand to ensure less tissue damage.
2. Choose a dentist or periodontist who uses ultrasonic tools and who does not remove layers of the cementum.
3. Insist that gum pockets be cleaned **only** if they are very inflamed or deeper than 4mm.
4. The dentist should be minimally invasive with their cleaning procedure. If an anesthetic is necessary, the treatment is likely too aggressive.[23]

Nutritional Reduction in Pocket Depth

Alvin Danenberg, DDS, and I collaborated in the summer of 2014 to study the effect of diet on gum disease.[24] Dr. Danenberg found that patients taking cod liver oil, butter oil, or skate liver oil along with kelp powder averaged 1.5mm reduction for pockets deeper than 6mm, and a 66 percent reduction in bleeding sites.[25] These improvements occurred over the course of thirty days with no other interventions. The average pocket reduction from scaling and root planing for similar sized pockets led to a 2.16mm in pocket reduction and 57 percent reduction in bleeding. *In other words, one month of basic nutritional therapy yielded results closely comparable to a scaling and root planing procedure.* It is reasonable to assume that a more prolonged or in-depth nutritional intervention could result in even more impressive results.

Gum Flap Surgery / Osseous Surgery

Traditional gum flap surgery involves cutting the gums open so the tooth root can be cleaned and the infected bone reshaped to reduce the pocket size. The dental surgeon removes infected tissue and remodels and smoothes the bone using a drill. Healing from the procedure is typically slow and often includes: post surgical pain, scar tissue formation, and gum recession of 2-4mm or more, along with sensitivity to cold food or drinks. You might wonder why this procedure is recommended when it causes so much gum recession? This is a good question for which I do not have a clear answer. However, the theory underlying traditional gum flap surgery is to surgically remove the infection and tighten up gum pockets to stabilize the supporting bone. This procedure is not only traumatic, but also yields unpredictable results. A more technologically advanced form of this surgery in now available called Minimally Invasive Periodontal Surgery. It employs a videoscope, allowing surgeons to make smaller and more specific incisions.[26]

How Effective Is Periodontal Surgery vs. Scaling and Root Planing?

A comprehensive review of longitudinal studies of treatment outcomes comparing scaling and root planing (SRP) procedures to traditional periodontal surgery found that results varied depending on the depth of the pockets.[27] SRP on gum pockets 4-6mm deep showed significantly more gum attachment gain than open flap surgery. However, gum flap surgery had more attachment gain than SRP when the pockets were greater than 6mm. This is presumably because it is more difficult to clean deposits in the larger, more inflamed, and degenerated pockets.

A study published in the *Journal of Periodontal Research* compared SRP to traditional gum flap surgery over a period of five years, and found that gum flap surgery resulted in a small loss in gum attachment while SRP resulted in a small gain.[28] Yet another study showed that SRP on 4-6 mm pockets resulted in 0.4mm more attachment gain than surgical therapy.[29]

Bone Replacement Grafts: The purpose of bone replacement grafts is to regenerate and promote bone formation. The gum is cut open and a bone matrix material is placed into the jaw bone to establish a matrix for new bone to grow and form.[30]

Guided Tissue Regeneration: This involves cutting open the gums and placing a membrane to protect the damaged tissue area and allow it to heal. The evidence shows that this treatment can reduce probing depth and lead to gum attachment gains more effectively than open flap surgery.[31]

Growth Factors

Various growth factors (such as IGF-1, FGF, TGF, and PDGF) can aid periodontal wound healing and regeneration.[32] Periodontists have types of bone matrix available with growth factors for bone grafts, but I am not aware of any specific topical growth factors available, even though there is evidence to support their use. Real bovine colostrum (the first milk produced after calving) contains growth factors. Placing organic colostrum (such as the one available at: traditionalfoods.org) on or near areas of gum recession may effectively speed gum tissue healing due to the delivery of growth factors directly to the area of injury.

Dental Implants

Dental implants are a risky business, because over time, some implant patients can develop chronic fatigue and other autoimmune problems. Periodontal complications are a strong possibility as well.[33] A five-year study reported that 56 percent of patients receiving implants developed peri-implantitis,[34] which is inflammation, infection, and ultimately destruction of bone around the implant. The rate of longer-term implant failure is probably much higher. People with a history of gum disease are more prone to peri-implantitis and implant loss than those without.[35]

The majority of implants used are made out of titanium. Placing metal directly into the jawbone can trigger an allergic reaction.[36] Over time, this continuous allergic reaction can cause or contribute to autoimmune diseases.[37]

There are many additional concerns about implants. Implants do not form a perfect seal between the implant and the gum tissues, and therefore debris from the mouth can leak and get stuck around the implants.[38] Since an implant is placed where an unhealthy tooth was extracted, often there could be a bone infection already developing where the implant is placed.[39] Minor bone infections can be hard to see on an X-ray. The implant crown is usually made from a different metal than the implant post, which creates a galvanic current.[40] Galvanic corrosion is the principle that batteries work on: when there are dissimilar metals in the presence of an electrolyte fluid, an electrical charge is created. When two different metals are in the mouth combined with saliva, the same thing happens that happens in a battery, and it is called dental galvanism.[41] It saddens and angers me that the dental field mostly ignores this simple scientific fact and observable phenomena. Additional metals besides the implant in the patient's mouth could exacerbate the problem.[42] (Note: dental crowns often are made with metals even if they appear white in color.) Teeth are normally supported by the flexible and elastic periodontal ligament. Implanted teeth lack elasticity as they are simply a metal post directly implanted in the jaw bone or upper palate, without any shock absorbing ability. Dental implants therefore may place abnormal stress or force at the implant site from biting or chewing.

Implants are not cheap. A single implant can cost from $4,000 to $5,000, and full mouth implants range from $30,000 to $80,000. I have been informed by other dentists that they have seen how the powerful profit potential of implants has led some dental practices to take a pessimistic view on saving teeth, because saving teeth generates less money than implants. I was old told that dental school education has much more focus on dental implants than ever before. Dentists may also justify the position of placing implants for vital teeth with the belief that since people's teeth will eventually fall out, which they often do as we age due to a demineralized diet, that it saves the patient money in the long run by getting an implant as soon as possible. I hope you can see the faulty logic with this position, especially in light of the nutritional information discussed in this book.

Zirconium implants are still considered experimental, but they are now FDA approved, and will likely prove to be a safer alternative to titanium implants.[43] Zirconia is a ceramic made from zirconium and its primary advantage over titanium is that it does not induce a galvanic current. Even with its possible advantages, this material does not solve the problem of gums not sealing to the implant surface and the problem of excessive pressure at the implant site. Consequently, infection or fracturing of the implant may occur over time.

Despite the risk factors of implants, which many patients are not clearly aware of, they are still a popular tooth replacement option because they provide a strong chewing surface and an aesthetic appeal. One advantage of implants is that having multiple implants stimulates the alveolar bone and thus slows down the rate of bone loss in the jaw because the biting pressure encourages bone remodeling and repair.

Laser Treatments for Gum Recession

Lasers are a promising new field for periodontal treatment. However the peer reviewed literature gives us contradictory information about the effectiveness of laser curettage. Several studies have reported that laser surgery is less painful and heals faster than traditional scalpel surgery.[44] However, another body of research suggests that lasers are accompanied by more pain and slower healing.[45]

Two meta-analyses of all studies regarding laser treatments clearly state that well designed studies proving the effectiveness of laser therapy is lacking.[46, 47] A meta-analysis of Nd:YAG laser for treatment of gum disease showed that they are not much more effective than the controls which were usually SRP.[48] Conversely, two studies reported treatments with the Nd:YAG laser showed some teeth built new cementum and that new connective tissue was forming. But not every tooth with the laser treatment healed this way—some healed via long junctional epithelial attachment, which is a form of healing but it does not resemble the original periodontal attachment.[49, 50] These two small laser studies showed that in about half of the treated teeth the laser treatment protocol helped reform the original connection between the tooth and gum, which is not a result found with the traditional gum flap surgery.

Laser curettage is not generally meant as a replacement for scaling and root planning (SRP).[51] Rather, laser treatment is indicated in combination with SRP for chronic periodontal disease with significant bony defects.[52, 53] In one study with eight patients suffering from chronic periodontal disease, 58 percent of the treated sites gained attachment, and 73 percent of the sites decreased in probing depth with the combination of laser curettage, and aggressive scaling and root planning.[54] The results for this study were substantially better than the average results for traditional gum flap surgery. The average tissue recession in this study was three-quarters a millimeter. Laser sterilization costs $250-$400 per session and complete full mouth periodontal treatment with a specific laser protocol can cost as much as $4,000 to $15,000.[55]

Cold laser therapy, also know as low-level laser therapy, uses light to stimulate the healing of body tissues. The correct choice of low-level laser frequencies and/or electrical impulses seems to aid the healing process of gum disease without incisions or curettage.

Anti-Bacterial Treatments

Many dentists recommend rinsing the mouth with anti-bacterial mouthwash as a treatment for gum disease. Anti-bacterial treatments give the gums an appearance of health, but the effects are only temporary.[56] Furthermore, it appears that it is the mechanical flushing of the pocket with fluid and not the antibiotics that reduces subgingival irritation.[57] Studies show that pharmaceutical antibiotics, antiseptics, and anti-inflammatory agents do not work as stand-alone procedures.[58] *These findings support the fact that gum disease is not a problem of bacterial invasion, but a problem of imbalanced body chemistry that is primarily due to a faulty diet.* Antibiotics in the mouth also contribute to the destruction of healthy bacteria in the digestive tract, possibly leading to future digestive disturbances and other health challenges.

Endoscopically Enhanced Scaling and Root Planing

The standard scaling and root planing (SRP) procedure is done blindly. Without the use of the newest available technology, dentists and hygienists cannot see under the gum line and so they just feel their way around with the scaling tool. As a result of the blind approach, tissues are more easily traumatized, patients experience more pain, and calculus and plaque are missed. It makes sense to use modern technology to see inside the gum pockets, yet most dentists do not offer this option. Seeing in the gum pocket can be done with an endoscope, which is a tiny medical camera designed for this purpose. Currently, perioendoscopic assisted scaling and root planing is more efficient and less invasive than scaling and root planing done without an endoscope.

An Example of Integrated Gum Disease Care

Regenerative Periodontal Endoscopy™ is a synergistic approach in which a naturopathic or medical doctor helps the patient to attain better health prior to perioendoscopic root debridement. Problems addressed prior to initiating oral treatment include systemic problems such as vitamin D and B12 deficiencies, anemia, diabetes, glandular imbalances, hormonal issues, autoimmune disorders, and systemic inflammation. During the perioendoscopic cleaning, regenerative proteins are placed on the cleaned tooth root surface to encourage regeneration. This integrated treatment method achieves superior results because it addresses the health of the entire patient and not just the symptoms of gum disease. You can learn more about this approach at periopeak.com

Occlusion and Gum Recession

The act of chewing creates a mighty force of seventy to five hundred pounds per square inch on our teeth. When this force is misplaced even slightly by a "bad bite," these pressures can easily accelerate alveolar bone destruction. The term used to describe this action is "occlusional trauma," and when there is trauma from occlusion, it can aggravate and inflame periodontal disease.[59] (Occlusion was also discussed at the end of chapter three.) A misplaced bite can be caused by bad orthodontics, poor dental work, or other injury to the body, head, or sacrum, such as a car accident. Misaligned bones, particularly in the head, or misaligned teeth can place pressure on the wrong teeth in the wrong places when engaged in the normal process of chewing, biting, or closing the mouth with teeth touching. (*Author's note*: Orthodontic treatments frequently damage the body, face, and periodontium; you can learn more about injuries caused by orthodontics and alternative palate expansion techniques at **curegumdisease.com/orthodontics**.)

Occlusion does not appear to be a primary factor in gum disease,[60] but when tissue destruction is already underway, a bad bite can accelerate and exacerbate the destruction. As a result, a bad bite (malocclusion) may slow down or even prevent natural healing from gum disease. One way this can happen is by increasing sympathetic dominance, the state of nervous system excitation commonly associated with gum disease.

The best way to resolve malocclusion is to look for the specific cause and address it directly, rather than make other changes to the bite to correct the compensation pattern. Typical sources of malocclusion include:

1. **Poor dental work**, namely fillings, inlays, crowns, and bridges that are too high or too low. Seemingly unrelated health issues can be a result of faulty dental work, including: TMJ (jaw) disorders, headaches, and painful teeth.
2. **Significant injuries** to other parts of the body. Given that the entire body is interconnected, even a foot injury could actually change someone's bite.
3. **Orthodontics** can lead to straight teeth but a bad bite, making you susceptible to bite-related gum problems. Braces usually force teeth into a certain configuration causing stress to the TMJ and alveolar bone. In combination with a less-than-optimal diet, over time, this can result in gum recession.[61]
4. **Dental procedures** themselves can cause a bad bite. Drilling teeth can cause teeth to rotate, lift up, or depress into the socket, making them too high, too low, or moving them into the wrong place. TMJ problems can result if the dentist pushes, pulls, leans on, or overstretches the jaw. Gum recession is most likely to occur at sites of faulty dental work.[62]
5. **Emotions** such as stress and depression can also place extra pressure on the bite. People who suppress their emotions can create tension in the head and jaw, which can eventually overstress the teeth.

In a healthy person, normal biting or clenching of the teeth is designed to rebalance and reset the eight cranial bones and fourteen facial bones automatically and help our body relax and realign. And any of the aforementioned conditions can interfere with this function, leading to malocclusion, which can result in increased gum recession.

Some dentists are aware of this bite issue, but struggle to fix the problem appropriately. For example, many dentists use a bite sensor or bite paper to measure the patient's bite, and then grind down tooth structure where the bite is out of balance. If done incorrectly, which happens a majority of the time,[63] it can lead to unexpected and seemingly unrelated future health challenges. Patients can develop lower back or knee pains, digestive problems, autoimmune disorders, chronic migraines, and many other ills from poor bite adjustments. By the same token, misalignments in the body can result in a poor bite, so grinding down teeth may often be addressing the problem at a symptomatic point and not at the source. Applied kinesiology testing, such as performed by a chiropractor, is one way to pinpoint the cause of the malocclusion, but extremely few dentists are trained in this skill.

A more enlightened approach seeks to unwind the original cause of the bite problem. For example, if a crown is too high or too low, it needs to be adjusted. However with a crown that is too high, the body has already adapted to the poor dental work and now, the teeth, the cranial bones, the facial bones, and likely other bones, muscles, and tendons in the body need to be adjusted before grinding down teeth should be even considered. Ill-fitting crowns are a common problem. One reason this happens is because crowns are fitted when patients are lying down in the dental chair. For a more accurate alignment, the patient's feet should be on the ground. Bite tests are most accurate when the entire body is in correct alignment and not fully reclined in the awkward dental chairs.

There are dentists who do resolve bite problems by trying to restore balance to the patient's entire body, particularly the skull bones, before trying to fix their teeth. Craniosacral therapy (learn more or find a practitioner at upledger.com) is a superior method for resolving issues in the nervous and skeletal systems. Pronated feet, old injuries, surgeries, scars, and misaligned cranial bones can all actually cause the bite to be off. Dedicated craniosacral practitioners can even unwind stress in the teeth, maxilla, jaw, and alveolar bone, usually imparting a great sense of relief to the patient. Chiropractors, osteopaths, and other body workers can also realign the body, head, and teeth. However, once a tooth has been drilled or ground down either as a method to balance the bite, or as a part of a dental treatment, it is very hard to correct or compensate for what has been done.

One solution to this dilemma is the Occlusal Cranial Balancing Technique,[64] which was developed to balance the bite without drilling down teeth. Very thin build-ups are placed on specific teeth while checking for motion and response in the cranial bones. As a result, natural tooth is not removed for the procedure.

Many people clench or grind their teeth at night, putting extra stress on the periodontium, which in turn speeds recession in people susceptible to gum disease. If you have bite-related problems, wearing night guards can be a temporary solution which allows your teeth and gums to rest at night while you investigate your next step. A night guard (without expansion screws) placed on the top teeth freezes the motion in the maxilla (upper palate) and distorts and cramps the essential cranial rhythm of the body. All of the bones in the head and face are designed to be mobile, almost as if they are breathing. A well-made night guard on the lower teeth can help the jaw find a more comfortable resting point without restricting the cranial rhythm. A well-made night guard can ease bite stress, relax the body and jaw joint, and facilitate deep and restful sleep and therefore healing.

Hidden Osteomyelitis / Osteonecrosis (Cavitations)

Hidden infections in the jaw could be classified as osteomyelitis lesions or osteonecrosis of the jaw. In layman's terms, they are often referred to as cavitations, which is short for NICO lesions (**N**euralgia-**I**nducing **C**avitational **O**steonecrosis). This phenomenon has largely been ignored by the medical profession, although it has been discussed in the dental literature over the past century.[65] Cavitations frequently occur at tooth extraction sites because a pocket or void is left in the jaw bone after the tooth is extracted. When the bone heals, it covers the small hole rather than fill it in, leaving a void of decreased circulation. Toxins are trapped in the small, now covered hole and those restricted tissues can more easily rot away. These are usually painless unless pressure is put on them, and they slowly release toxins into the body.

Hidden infections in your body can be from old surgeries and injuries that do not heal correctly. But the most common source of hidden infections in the body is right in our heads. The sites of tooth extractions, including wisdom teeth, are often infected but undiagnosed. Root canals are also frequently infected, and just as with tooth extraction sites, these infections are difficult or impossible to see on an X-ray. Other causes of hidden infections in the jaw bone are a physical injury, jaw surgery, or bite interferences. Hidden infections in the mouth can lead to poor digestion, sympathetic dominance, and even spread disease to other parts of the body that seem completely unrelated.[66] When infective substances from the mouth leak to other parts of the body, they can contribute to inflammatory conditions such as arthritis.[67] Having symptoms on one side of the body can often be a sign of a hidden infection on the same side of the body in the mouth. For example, having a bad left shoulder and a healthy right shoulder could indicate a problem on the left side of the mouth.

One way to check for hidden infections is with pH paper. If your urine is generally more alkaline than your saliva, it almost always means there is an infection.[68] Hidden infections significantly contribute to acidic pH values and imbalanced body chemistry. Healing the infection makes it much easier for the whole body to heal and find balance.

Clearing Cavitations

Non-surgical treatments for cavitations include ozone injections, low level laser, frequency machines,[69] calcium chips, homeopathy, and massaging essential oils into the gums. Some dentists who clean out cavitations say that it is impossible to fully heal them without surgery.[70] Even if surgery is required, performing non-invasive treatments beforehand could help reduce the level of infection and irritation prior to the surgery. The least invasive form of surgery is to clean out the infection with hand tools (not a dental drill) and to sterilize the infection using ozonated magnesium chloride.[71] Cavitation surgery must be performed very carefully, as it is easy to damage nerves in the mouth.

The at-home treatment for cavitations is something that is both safe to do, and if you have ever had extractions (including wisdom teeth), I would recommend you try this essential oil program for one to two weeks as it may aid your healing process.

Choose one essential oil from each category and rotate oils from each category either throughout the day, the week, or the month. To apply, the essential oil is usually too strong and needs to be diluted into a cold pressed carrier oil such as almond oil, sunflower, or olive oil. The approximate ratio is six drops of essential oil for one tablespoon of carrier oil.[72] (This mixture would be enough for many applications.) Apply the mixed oil on your finger and massage it on your gums at points of infection or tooth extraction. For whole body balancing, rub the oil on the bottom of your feet. Apply the oil twice per day, or more often if convenient.

Category A (phenols): wintergreen, anise, birch, clove, and basil.

Category B (sesquiterpenes): black pepper, patchouli, German chamomile, cedarwood, sandalwood, myrrh, and frankincense.

Category C (monoterpenes): grapefruit, silver fir, bitter orange, mandarin, and orange.

Essential oils can be purchased online or at a local health food store, though bear in mind that not all are the same quality, and if you are pregnant or nursing some essential oils are contraindicated.[73]

Calcium Therapy

The primary cause of gum disease is calcium and other minerals precipitating out of the periodontium as a result of low blood calcium,[74] which is primarily from vitamins and minerals lacking in the diet. It therefore makes sense that a topical calcium therapy might help in treating gum disease.

Calcium therapy has achieved good results both in patients' homes and in the dental office for gum disease.[75] Unlike treatment with harsh chemicals, calcium therapy enhances the host response in the mouth by adding calcium to the inflamed tissues.[76] Office treatments offer better support and precision than in-home treatments. For a home calcium therapy kit, or a referral for non-surgical gum disease treatment, visit **calciumtherapy.com**.

Evidence-Based Care

It is the legal, ethical, and moral obligation of each dentist to incorporate new scientific evidence into his or her standard of care, and to provide informed consent for the treatment prescribed. Informed consent means that permission is granted for the treatment by the patient with the full knowledge of the possible consequences and risks of the treatment. In this chapter I have presented some of the literature in relation to the effectiveness of gum disease treatments. Dentists often do not incorporate the newest evidence to improve how they treat their patients in the office. As a result, patients are deprived of the most effective treatments which they deserve to be offered.

The Bigger Picture about Healing Gum Disease

As has been stated, gum disease is a symptom of an imbalance in the entire body, caused primarily by nutrient deficiencies. Because surgeries and local treatments do not treat the root cause of gum disease,[77] patients who rely solely on periodontal treatments unfortunately continue to lose their teeth.[78]

Because the majority of the evidence suggests that the host response is the essential factor in whether one succumbs to periodontal disease or remains immune to it, any treatment that fails to address the person's overall health does not completely serve the patient. Neglecting the true cause of periodontal disease allows it to continue and often get worse. When it gets worse and patients do not recover, it creates a scenario where more dental treatments are needed. Sadly, the patient losing their teeth, and their hard earned dollars, means that dentists make more money and have more patients. This dynamic creates a perverse incentive which stifles innovation and truly curative treatments from being brought into the dental profession. Probably from fear, dentists rarely discuss problems that they experience in dentistry, and this lack of conversation stifles change and awareness and allows things to continue as they are.

How Dentistry Needs to Change to Serve Humanity

If dentists listened to their own intuition in observing their patients and availed themselves to the evidence presented in this book regarding nutrition therapies, dentists today might once again become the courageous leaders for health and change, and walk in the footsteps of dentists who truly healed their patients like doctors Price, Page, and Hawkins. The great religions of the world, along with many indigenous traditions, believe that the spirit of service to others is a primary human and spiritual value. Until dental professionals embrace this concept of service, and embody it by advocating and practicing the least invasive and most holistic treatment paradigms, dentistry in general will continue to hurt people by cutting and poisoning when it is not needed.

Conventional dental treatments that eliminate pocket depth, re-contour the bones, and scour teeth, do not provide a long-term or systemic cure. Neglecting patients by treating surface symptoms and not causes is a form of passive harm. The field of periodontology was designed to treat unhealthy people who are essentially malnourished, and who have succumbed to poor dietary habits. The system is run by practitioners who in general do not eat well and who are not in peak health themselves; therefore, their conclusions about gum disease are based in part on their personal experiences. By significantly improving one's diet, many of the current rules and expectations of conventional treatment outcomes no longer apply.

The historical literature has pointed again and again to the fact that gum disease is a whole body health problem. When people face gum disease, they go to the dentist. But they receive only specialized treatment focused on oral tissues, and the condition of the rest of the body is ignored. I advocate for the field of dentistry to include prevention of disease as well as whole body treatments by embracing information on body chemistry, cranial work, and nutrition. This would be a big leap for the profession since these areas are not taught in standard dental schools. Furthermore, professional partnerships can also be formed where dentists work with naturopaths, craniosacral therapists, osteopaths, and the like to enrich the field and expand the range of successful therapies available to patients. I would like to see all of this not only legally sanctioned, but also encouraged.

Unfortunately I have heard many shocking stories of dentists and doctors losing their licenses for trying to help people with holistic treatments. Some states are better than others in this regard, but today in many locations in the United States, there are still the "witch hunts" of darker times happening. So-called "alternative" doctors and dentists are expelled from the field for trying something different and for speaking out, as I am, against the stagnant and life-negating status quo. Because of these modern day "witch hunts," many dentists are afraid to honestly speak their mind, and they share what they really feel and know only in private. The unfortunate result is that the industry stays repressed and frozen, and in the end, patients do not receive the real, lasting, and nourishing care that they deserve.

Toward a Less Invasive Treatment Model

The whole model of dentistry has changed from what it used to be. Dentists are now like oral plastic surgeons. There is little or no thought of the physiology and biochemistry going on **underneath the surface** which causes gum disease. With serious illnesses like gum disease, our bodies are frequently imbalanced because they are poisoned by heavy metals, chemicals, pesticides, hidden infections, and vaccine toxins. Cleansing and supporting the functions of the liver, kidneys, and other organs helps the body to heal and utilize food efficiently.

Educating dentists about holistic treatments can be transformative and life-changing if they are open to the idea. Both dentists and their patients will benefit from an enlightened approach to dental care that is informed by a philosophy of love, nurturance, and respect for the body and an emphasis on less dental treatments, and more emphasis on a whole body approach.

More enlightened dentistry would include:

1. Preparing the body for days, weeks, or even months with nutrition and body chemistry balancing before doing even one treatment so that the body heals properly.
   a. Using systemic treatments including metabolic typing diets, and specifically targeted dietary supplements.
   b. Healing and cleansing the digestive system and body by aiding elimination and detoxification mechanisms in the body.
2. Regular checkups that include monitoring body chemistry using non-invasive methods to control and prevent tooth decay and gum disease before it occurs.

Dentist Melvin Page believed that not only could dentists prevent dental decay (and gum disease), but that they could do far more: "a dentist, by testing for susceptibility to dental decay and treating the patient to produce immunity can prevent and cure other degenerative diseases."[79]

What to Expect from Nutritional Healing of Gum Disease

There have been reports that with significant dietary and health changes very deep gum pockets—as deep as 10mm—can heal.[80] After correcting your diet—over a period of several months—red, swollen, and tender gums should decrease or go away entirely. Bleeding from probing, flossing, or eating hard food should continually reduce until there is no more bleeding. Gums will no longer pull away from your teeth and loose teeth will become firmly implanted. Bad breath should turn to acceptable breath and in the ideal situation, turn into pleasant breath. Most importantly, you will feel better.

This happens when, over time, bone density significantly increases and the periodontal ligament repairs itself from diet. This does not mean that where there is a complete absence of alveolar bone that it can grow back, but rather, any tiny bit of bone left can substantially harden and fill in, and remaining ligaments and tissues can strengthen. If the alveolar bone has been totally destroyed, it cannot likely be regrown without some type of grafting material to create a scaffold for new bone growth. Even in those cases, balancing body chemistry with a good diet will significantly hasten and improve any surgical outcome.

If you have massive gum tissue loss in which your gum line has migrated substantially down the tooth, it isn't likely that you will have the tissue return too much, even with an excellent diet. But you can expect the improvements in diet to halt your gum tissue degeneration, and for your teeth to become more firmly rooted in place. Furthermore, even people with no teeth still suffer from bone loss in their jaw, making implants fail, and dentures loose and uncomfortable. In other words, *nobody can escape gum recession unless they make real changes to improve their diet.*

Because gum tissues will become firmer and stronger, some readers will be able to avoid dental treatment entirely. Others will be able to get by with just one gentler scaling and root planing, and never see calculus or gum recession again.

A portion of readers, perhaps between 5-15 percent, will struggle to properly digest and assimilate food well enough to balance their body chemistry to stop gum disease. For those, you will likely need to seek additional help, such as from a functional medicine practitioner, naturopathic doctor, or other alternative practitioner to further help hone in on the body chemistry solution to your gum disease. Even for these difficult cases, this book may still serve as an eye-opening guide to help clarify the true nature of gum disease and point you in the right direction as to how to heal your condition.

Creating a Treatment Plan to Cure Gum Disease Naturally

I hope the message of this chapter and book is clear. No matter what treatment option you choose for yourself, you will only enjoy long-term healing when you change both your diet and lifestyle.

Only you can decide which treatment is right for you. Since everyone is different and every situation is unique, there is no "one size fits all" approach. That is why I tried to give you the clearest information I could find, without giving an exact recommendation about what you should do, so you can come to rational decisions on your own.

The challenge of designing your treatment program is getting the right amount of help. There are two sides of the coin when it comes to periodontal and health professionals. Some health professionals can be overbearing, controlling, demanding, and might coerce you to accept treatments that you do not need or want. They may also make promises to help you and then not really have remedies for your specific situation, leaving you disheartened. Conversely, entirely avoiding professional help could lead to your missing out on useful therapies that might help you. Understand that each approach has its perils, proceed with confidence and a desire to educate yourself, so that you will make the best decisions for yourself.

In the end, choosing good treatments means taking care of yourself in a loving way. Ask yourself what truly honoring and loving yourself really looks like? Take a moment and think about, and preferably write down what are your real needs, desires, and hopes in relation to gum disease. What you want and need is vital and not to be ignored or stuffed away. The more you can connect with what you really want and need, the more empowered you will be to find outer support, or perhaps feel confident in the do-it-yourself approach. Only you know what is right. Some treatment methods are better than others, but in the end, you have to make the final decision on whom to trust and what to do. I wish you every success in this endeavor.

Again, *only you can decide which treatment is right for you.* Yes, I am repeating this point, but it is an important reminder that I want you to take to heart. No matter what treatment option you choose, know you will get the best long-term results when you change your diet and how you live. Here are just a few ideas of what some different treatment paths could look like considering the keystone of nutrition.

A Home Approach to Cure Gum Disease – Example Treatment Outline

1. Align your vision of health and really think and feel into what you need and want (discussed in chapter seven).

2. Support your overall health and digestion (also discussed in chapter seven).
3. Improve diet as described in this book.
4. Use gum and mouth cleaning suggestions from the next chapter.
5. Utilize supportive treatments like herbal medicine, acupuncture, craniosacral, and chiropractic care.
6. Monitor progress with a journal or photographs, keeping track of disease symptoms like bleeding, loose teeth, or inflammation.

A Gentle Holistic Approach that Combines Dietary Changes with a Professional Treatment – Example Treatment Outline

1. Align your vision of health and really think and feel into what you need and want (discussed in chapter seven).
2. Support your overall health and digestion (also discussed in chapter seven).
3. Improve your diet for two to four weeks and practice gentle and holistic home care as discussed in the next chapter.
4. Gentle root cleaning with a dentist or periodontist you trust on specific sites where needed.
5. Monitor the progress and healing both in the dental office and at home by taking notes of your symptoms, while continuing to eat a healthy diet.
6. If your body chemistry returns to balance, no more deep cleanings would be needed and office visits would just be maintenance and checkups.

Ample Support for Severe Gum Disease Holistic Treatment – Example Treatment Outline

1. Align your vision of health and really think and feel into what you need and want (discussed in chapter seven).
2. Create your support team to include a dentist or periodontist, along with at least one holistic whole body health practitioner.
    a. Find a trusted holistic practitioner such as a naturopath, acupuncturist, functional medicine doctor, or chiropractor, to get excellent support with a specific diet just right for you, along with cleansing and detoxification, and specific help with supplements to take for your specific imbalances. *You may need more than one practitioner to help you.*
    b. Find a dental specialist who offers treatments you feel interested in. Evaluate the different treatment options with your health care team and consider them carefully.

3. Consider structural or protective treatments like night guards, and consider ways to carefully reduce stress on teeth such as with craniosacral or osteopathic treatments.
4. Have the chosen treatment performed and monitor progress with your integrative care team while staying on a healthy diet.

Chapter 9 Summary – Dentistry and Gum Disease

- ☐ Dental trauma and abuse happens when we have treatments pushed upon us that are unnecessary or that we did not fully consent to.
- ☐ Gum disease is a nutritional problem and has little to do with bacteria. Since most of the justification of treatments is to get rid of the bacteria or their results, it is possible that entire portions of the conventional treatment paradigm are flawed because they are not based in reality.
- ☐ Take care to find a dentist, hygienist, or periodontist that you feel good about. These practitioners will give you a sense of well-being and you will feel good visiting with them. If you feel unsure of any treatment prescribed, take the time to get more informed before moving forward.
- ☐ Overtreatment is common in the field of dentistry which means that patients should be cautious before consenting to any significant treatment.
- ☐ Scaling and root planing is the standard conventional method of treating gum disease. It should be tried before any surgery is recommended.
- ☐ Nutrition may reduce pocket depths as much or more than scaling and root planing.
- ☐ Dental implants are prone to infections and cause galvanic currents, make sure you understand the risks of implants before choosing them.
- ☐ Laser treatments may be better than gum flap surgery.
- ☐ Anti-bacterial treatments do not work and may not be necessary.
- ☐ New technology can assist in more precise scaling and root planing.
- ☐ Occlusion is a factor in gum recession that needs to be paid attention to, but it is not a cause by itself.
- ☐ Hidden infections can interfere with the body's healing and create acidity in the body from poor digestion.
- ☐ Calcium therapy is a non-invasive treatment protocol for gum disease.
- ☐ It is time for dentistry to change and consider a whole body approach for tooth decay and gum disease.

10 Natural Gum Care at Home

When healing your gums with diet, it is still useful to manage the symptoms of gum disease with proper gum care. Brushing and flossing are often not enough to give the mouth an extra boost when dealing with infection or inflammation from gum disease. While many of the methods discussed in this chapter might be considered alternative or experimental, some scientific evidence, along with plenty of people's experience, supports their use.

Sea Salt Mouthwash for Gum Disease

Author of *Money by the Mouthful,* Robert Nara, DDS, recommends regularly rinsing the mouth with a sea salt solution. While treating gum disease as a dentist in the military, he found this easy and inexpensive method improved and sometimes even cured his patients' gum disease.[1]

Sea salt water mouthwash is fast and simple. At least twice per day, morning and night, rinse with warm salt water. Mix one-half to one teaspoon of salt with one cup of warm water. Swish the warm salt water around in your mouth for thirty to sixty seconds. That's it!

Sea salt water rinse is more effective with an oral irrigator. Keep in mind that salt water use will void the warranty and shorten the lifespan of your oral irrigation device. To minimize the damage caused by salt, run a full reservoir of plain water through after each use.

Water Flossing for Gum Disease

To "water floss," you'll need a device such as ViaJet Pro®, Waterpik®, or Hydro Floss®. These oral irrigators reach places that regular flossing cannot. The pulsation of the water from these devices helps stimulate the gums and thereby improve circulation. These oral irrigators are designed by their manufacturers to be used with plain water only. However, their healing power is enhanced if essential oils, herbal tinctures, baking soda, and/or sea salt are added to the water in the irrigators. For this reason, alternative medicine practitioners and some dentists recommend a variety of gum healing substances be added to the irrigator before using. In particular, herbal tinctures can be both soothing and medicinal to inflamed gums.

While these techniques are therapeutic and I think many readers will benefit from using them, you should know that all of these uses will void the irrigator warranty and shorten its lifespan. The stronger or higher concentration the oil, the more damage it can cause. Diluting essential oils or sea salt in a separate vessel and then pouring them in the irrigator reservoir can reduce sediment build-up and reduce the likelihood of damage. Even so, people who use salt or essential oils usually end up needing to replace their irrigators with some regularity. If that becomes too expensive, a manual syringe-style irrigator can serve as an oral irrigator. Very deep pockets may require a pocket syringe to irrigate them.

Make sure to review the directions of your oral irrigator. It is possible to push the toxins from the gum pocket into the blood stream if wrongly used.

Tooth Brushing with Toothpaste

Toothpaste originally evolved out of tooth polish made from chalk or pumice. Much like polishing shoes, it was done on occasion to shine up and whiten the teeth. It was not originally a twice-a-day routine. This all changed in the early 1900s when Claude Hopkins, author of *Scientific Advertising,* decided to market Pepsodent® dentifrice. To build demand for this product, he had to first create a desire in people to brush their teeth. Though he had no evidence whatsoever, Hopkins warned consumers that they needed to brush every day to prevent gum disease, keep their teeth clean, and have a beautiful white smile.[2] He was so successful that other toothpaste companies soon followed Pepsodent®, and in fact, overtook it as market leaders.

Today the average toothpaste is still based somewhat upon the Pepsodent® formula. Toothpastes are usually composed of 20-60 percent abrasive and polishing compounds, and 20-40 percent moisture-retaining substances such as glycerin, sorbitol, and propylene glycol. The remaining 1-2 percent consists of preservatives, sweeteners, dyes, fluoride, antibiotics, binders, detergents, and fragrances.[3] Some of the substances added to commercial toothpastes are essentially toxic or poisonous, such as fluoride. Other substances added are not natural and generally do not support whole body health, such as industrial-made sweeteners like glycerin or xylitol. My philosophy with tooth cleaning is that if you would not eat or swallow the ingredients, you probably should not be putting it in your mouth.

Because most toothpaste is abrasive,[4] it is easy to brush too hard and cause either tooth erosion or gum recession. One epidemiological study looking at toothpaste and tooth wear found that abrasive toothpaste definitely causes dentin wear,[5] and if it can wear your teeth, then it can wear down your gums. Another study found that hard brushing over time increased the likelihood of receded gum sites.[6] A medium or hard bristle toothbrush—in combination with the abrasive substances commonly found in most toothpastes—will lead to removal of enamel and gum recession in people whose body chemistry is out of balance.[7] This makes it important to use a soft bristle brush and take care with your choice of tooth cleaning products. When people are healthy and their body is in balance, hard tooth brushing and abrasive toothpastes can cause less damage, or the damage can repair itself, leading to some skepticism or denial by the dental community regarding the harm of hard toothbrushes or abrasive pastes.

Soft Toothbrushes Are Best for Improved Gum Health

Toothbrush hardness depends on bristle thickness. Thicker bristles will be stiffer. Soft toothbrushes have the thickness of seven mil (seven thousands of an inch) or less. Ultrasoft brushes such as for extremely sensitive gums are five mil and thinner. Medium bristle brushes are eight mil and up to twelve mil thick. Fourteen mil or thicker are considered hard brushes.[8] Given that tooth brushing can irritate the gums and wear away enamel, I recommend soft bristle brushes.[9] Toothbrushes should be replaced often, especially when you are susceptible to gum disease, as they collect dead skin cells and food remnants. Consider replacing your brush as often as once a month, and also consider regularly cleaning your toothbrush with warm water and a bit of soap.

Electric Toothbrushes

Electric toothbrushes seem to help some people with the healing of gum disease. But not all electric toothbrushes are good to use. As with regular toothbrushes, they should be very gentle and not irritate or abrade the gums. As I personally do not use one, I am of little help in recommending a specific brand or instructions for how to use them in relation to gum disease. But I am mentioning it here, because should

Gum Disease and Oral Health Tip: Clean Your Tongue

Tongue scraping helps improve bad breath, helps your mouth maintain its balance of pH and oral flora, enhances your ability to taste, and improves digestive health. You can clean your tongue by brushing it with your toothbrush. The traditional method of using a metal tongue scraper may be even more effective.

you feel inspired to get an electric tooth brush as part of your gum disease home care, a good choice might help you feel better.

Herbs for Gum Disease

Herbal products can help fight gum disease whether used internally, externally, or both.

White Oak Bark Powder has a reputation for strengthening gum tissues, though it may not help with receding gums. To use as a gum powder, apply a modest amount to the inflamed areas on the gums and leave it on overnight. Continue until the problem resolves.

Echinacea is a native herb traditionally used for the treatment of sore mouth and gum conditions. Although it is most often taken as a tea, the fresh root can be applied to a tooth for a toothache.[10] Echinacea is also a blood purifier. To use topically, place echinacea root powder on the inflamed area, or use approximately one dropper full of echinacea tincture with water as a tea or as a mouthwash.

Goldenseal is highly valued for helping digestive problems when taken orally,[11] as well as for strengthening the immune system. Goldenseal powder can be rubbed on the gums to treat gum disease. A powder or tincture can also be mixed with water and used as a mouthwash.

Myrrh Gum is an ancient healing herb, its use predating the Bible. It has a long history as a sovereign remedy for gum disease. Myrrh powder makes an excellent tooth powder and can ease inflammation and gum infections.[12] Myrrh tincture can be diluted with water and used as a mouthwash.

Chamomile tea or tincture can be used as a gargle or mouthwash for treating gingivitis.

Watercress is an ancient leafy green vegetable. Chewing watercress may make teeth stronger as well as help bleeding gums and gingivitis.

Prickly Ash Bark is the first ingredient in Edgar Cayce's famous tooth and gum formula Ipsab. Prickly ash bark helps improve circulation in the mouth and it creates a tingly sensation. It can also be used to treat toothache. Ipsab is available in many health food stores.

And *Herbal Tooth Powder* that contains many of the gum-healing herbs just mentioned is available traditionalfoods.org. It is very gentle and non-abrasive.

Herbal Precaution: Most people respond well to herbal tooth powders and poultices. People suffering from advanced periodontal disease with inflamed pockets, however, *might* experience irritation if tiny specks of herbs are left in the mouth. These people may wish to try liquid herbal products.

Baking Soda for Brushing and Whitening

Sodium bicarbonate is often promoted as a natural tooth powder. It is obviously cheap, and it is known for its alkalizing ability. Because most people with significant gum disease have an acidic pH, brushing with baking soda may be of benefit. Unfortunately baking soda does not work for everyone and it is not my personal preference to use it regularly. Baking soda can be too abrasive even though toothpastes are five to ten times more abrasive.[13] Baking soda is most useful as a tooth polish or whitener. Rubbing baking soda on stained teeth that have a translucent appearance can bring their whiteness back.

Toothpaste Alternatives

Many toothpastes, even "natural" ones, are abrasive to the teeth. Like toothpastes, many tooth powders are also too abrasive, so you need to be careful to choose a non-abrasive one. Abrasive pastes and powders leave teeth with a subtle irritated or itchy feeling. When you ditch the abrasive paste, sometimes there is a side effect of teeth appearing slightly stained or translucent due to a thin natural film remaining on the teeth. This film appears when the body chemistry is somewhat out of balance. If this happens to you, using baking soda on occasion can keep your teeth white.

There are a few good alternatives to toothpastes. And again, it is up to you to choose which ones you like, if any. Different people will have their favorites, as we are all unique. Find what works best for you. Some of the options out there are:

- ❑ Brushing with herbal tooth powder.
- ❑ Brushing with plain water (yes, I mean just water and nothing else!)
- ❑ Brushing with sea salt.
- ❑ Brushing with baking soda.
- ❑ Brushing with soap—this could be a clean bar of soap (like Dr. Bronner's) or a liquid soap product that is designed for the teeth.
- ❑ Brushing with essential oils.

For high quality tooth powder, mouthwash, and essential oil products visit traditionalfoods.org.

Traditional Cultures and Tooth Brushing

Those familiar with the work of Dr. Price as well as with traditional societies might know that some cultures who were healthy and free from tooth decay did not brush their teeth. Different traditional cultures around the world have different tooth care habits. Some use a natural tree resin chewing gum (tree resin gums are available at traditionalfoods.org), while others use sticks to clean their teeth. While I think most people will benefit from tooth brushing provided it is not too abrasive, some people have been able to get their body chemistry to such a balance that they have good breath and no deposits without any brushing at all.

Proxy Brushes are disposable little brushes that are used like flexible toothpicks between the teeth. They help remove food debris and plaque and are widely used by people with braces and bridges who cannot easily floss. Proxy brushes can also be useful for people with gum recession.[14] Get your brush wet and gently insert it into the gap between your teeth. Move the brush in and out gently. Do not use too much force and make sure to get both the lip side and tongue side of the tooth. For more instructions ask your dentist, hygienist, or review a video on YouTube.com.

Gum Massage

Try this right now. It is easy to massage your gums through your cheek, or by placing a finger directly in your mouth. Connect with the gum tissue, apply a bit of pressure, and slowly rub in small circles both clockwise and counterclockwise to bring healing and circulation to the area. If you are trying to clear an infection, gum massage can be done with essential oils either through the cheek or in the mouth. Essential oils good for healing gum tissue were discussed in chapter nine in the section on cavitations. Essential oils should be mixed with a carrier oil like sesame, almond, or olive oil.

The Taboo Mouthwash

Pierre Fauchard (1678 – 1761), considered the father of modern dentistry, believed that the dentifrices and mouthwashes of his time paled in comparison to a "natural" mouthwash that could whiten teeth and strengthen the gums: fresh urine.[15]

Oil Pulling for Oral Health

The ancient traditional Ayurvedic practice of "oil pulling" can pull embedded toxins out of the oral tissues, tighten the gums, and whiten the teeth. Oil pulling can be done up to three times a day on an empty stomach. Here's how:

- ☐ Upon waking and before eating or drinking, put approximately one tablespoon of cold-pressed coconut oil or sesame oil into your mouth.
- ☐ Swish and pull the oil around your mouth and through your teeth for fifteen to twenty minutes. While this length of time is ideal, many people cannot do it that long, so start out with whatever length of time is comfortable for you.
- ☐ **Important:** Do not swallow the oil. Its purpose is to collect toxins.
- ☐ Spit the oil into a lined garbage can or outside on the ground; do not spit into a sink or toilet where the accumulated oil might clog the drainage or septic system.
- ☐ Rinse with water twice.
- ☐ Brush your teeth.

Traditional Ayurvedic doctors recommend sesame oil for oil pulling because of its healing properties. Coconut oil also has strong antimicrobial and antibacterial properties. Today high quality coconut oil is more available than high quality, cold pressed sesame oil. Both oils work well and many "oil pullers" like to alternate between the two oils. Many people notice that their mouths feel cleaner and fresher even after their first time of practicing the procedure.

Possible Contraindication for Oil Pulling: A common symptom of mercury toxicity is bleeding gums and loose teeth.[16] Be cautious about frequent oil pulling with mercury fillings as the oil may release mercury. If you have mercury fillings, oil pulling may not be a good idea.

Avoid Commercial Mouthwashes

Antiseptic mouthwashes can be useful for acute oral infections, but their value for chronic infections is questionable.[17] Normal saliva is more effective at balancing oral flora than chemicals,[18] and constantly sterilizing the mouth does not help the body find microbial balance. To balance one's mouth, it is best to focus on nutritional and other natural therapies such as those discussed in this chapter and the rest of the book. Swishing with chemicals not only affects the mouth, but also the entire digestive tract, and can contribute to other health problems over time by killing off all the good bacteria.

Be Kind to Your Gums

It is important when you have gum disease or are susceptible to it to treat your gums gently to optimize your chances for healing. Watch out for these behaviors:

- ☐ **Aggressive tooth brushing and flossing** can cause damage to gum tissue.[19] Use a soft bristle toothbrush and do not apply large amounts of force while brushing.
- ☐ **Hot foods and drinks** can cause minor burns to the gum tissue.[20] Do not eat or drink foods that are overly hot. That means foods that create a burning sensation on your tongue.
- ☐ **Eating very hard, crunchy foods** or foods with small particles may inflame sensitive gum tissues.[21] Some examples of foods that could aggravate gums are potato chips, nuts, or bread with a very hard, crunchy crust.

- ☐ Do not get **new mercury fillings**, because mercury is toxic to your body and oral tissues.
- ☐ The topical application of fluoride can contribute to gingivitis and gum disease.[22] Avoid fluoridated drinking water and bathing water as well, because fluoride exposure is linked to increased incidence of gum disease (see chapter six for additional information).

Blotting Out Gum Disease

J.E. Phillips, DDS (1922-2003), was a forward-thinking dentist who believed plaque and tartar were symptoms of gum disease and not the cause. In his 1972 book, *Acquiring and Maintaining Oral Health,* he described a remarkable gum cleaning technique called "blotting," which he recommended for maintaining and restoring gum health. Unfortunately his theory never quite took off with the dental establishment, although there are a few dentists who still know about it and teach it to their patients because it is very effective.

Dr. Phillips believed bacteria were the "helpful watch dogs" of the mouth and that they are needed to prevent the growth of molds and fungus.[23] In other words, bacteria are present because they are eating away and cleaning up potentially more toxic substances formed in the body like mold and fungus.

Ahead of his time, in 1972, Dr. Phillips correctly identified plaque, the unwanted buildup of dead cells in the mouth,[24] and not calculus as the symptom that correlates with gum disease. When the plaque is removed, healing often begins.[25]

Dr. Phillips was convinced that normal tooth brushing jams the plaque into the gum crevice, where enzymes from the plaque attempt to break it down and in the process cause gum tissue destruction.[26] Dr. Phillips was opposed to the regular use of antibiotic chemicals, as he believed that most bacteria in the mouth are beneficial.[27] *It thus makes sense to clean the gums carefully after brushing with a gum cleaning brush or an oral irrigator.*

Cleaning Your Gums at Home

Dr. Phillips reported most people saw noticeable results from using his blotting technique within three weeks. This technique is optimally performed using brushes designed by Dr. Phillips himself. These are brushes whose bristles are made more porous through a texturizing process; however, I would expect for people on a budget that any soft bristle toothbrush will yield acceptable, but probably not optimal results. Dr. Phillips' technique works by tapping the special toothbrush at a forty-five degree angle into the gum crevice to suck up the plaque. To buy gum cleaning brushes that can also be used as regular soft bristle brushes and to watch instructional videos, visit curegumdisease.com/gumcleaning.

Dr. Phillips also noted that the teeth only represent a small part of the entire tissues in the mouth. Therefore, if we merely brush our teeth while ignoring all the other tissues, the mouth is really not being properly cleaned. During your normal twice-daily mouth cleaning routine, Dr. Phillips recommended that the soft bristle brush be brushed everywhere in the mouth and not just on the teeth. That means lightly rubbing your brush on the inside and outside of the gums, on all parts of the tongue including the back of the tongue, the roof of your mouth, the floor of your mouth, and your cheeks.

Chapter 10 Summary—Natural Gum Care

When healing your gums with diet, it is still useful to manage the symptoms of gum disease with proper gum care. Brushing and flossing are often not enough to give the mouth an extra boost when dealing with infection or inflammation from gum disease.

Try any or several of these mouth-cleaning concepts:

- ☐ Use an oral irrigator with warm water and sea salt.
- ☐ Practice oil pulling with sesame or coconut oils.
- ☐ Use an herbal gum powder or herbal mouthwash to soothe oral tissues.
- ☐ Avoid anti-bacterial mouthwashes and commercial mouthwashes.
- ☐ Be gentle with your mouth—aggressive tooth brushing, hot foods and drinks, and eating very hard, crunchy food can all irritate or damage sensitive gum tissues.
- ☐ Brush with a soft bristle brush.
- ☐ There are a number of herbs that may be beneficial for gum disease: white oak bark powder, echinacea, goldenseal, myrrh gum, chamomile, watercress, and prickly ash bark.
- ☐ Use Dr. Phillips' technique for cleaning gums.
- ☐ Avoid fluoridated water and fluoride treatments.
- ☐ Avoid abrasive toothpastes. Instead, use gentle herbal tooth powder, essential oils,
- ☐ sea salt, or baking soda.

Cure Gum Disease Naturally – Conclusion

Life is more than just a set of days to live out. Life is meant to be lived *through* you. As a culture, we have unknowingly accepted many practices generated by the field of dentistry that are not enlivening. We have put up with treatments that do not address the root cause of gum disease, and we have ignored great teachers like dentists Weston Price, Melvin Page, and Harold Hawkins, who paved the path toward real gum health. I have summarized and clarified their work in combination with up-to-date research and my own personal experience with oral health so that you can have the information you need to cure gum disease naturally.

The choice is now yours. Will you continue to accept a fate in which you have little control over your health? Will you submit the responsibility for your gum health to a professional who will make a profit from providing you a service that does not address the root of your disease? Or will you choose a new way of freedom and empowerment, in which you are completely responsible for your health, and can choose to turn to professionals when you need them to support you on your own healing journey?

There is so much more to life than suffering from poor health. But poor health stands in the way of us truly living and being in the world the way we want to be. It is time to let go of this outmoded way of living and being. For the dental profession, that means serving people first and placing patient health paramount to financial gain. For you, it means taking care of yourself: to follow that forgotten dream, to really reach out for what you need in life, to take a risk and to "bite" into life.

The industry of dentistry, as a collective, has unconsciously taken away our right for good oral health, and doing so increases dentists' profits, as people need more treatments and more severe treatments. Likewise, we have given it to them because in general, people have not been willing to face real responsibly for their health and/or are not aware of alternatives. The way we live our lives on a daily basis either contributes to our health or takes away from our health based on the choices we make. So regaining our gum health will involve changing our lifestyle.

Your health is both your right and your responsibility. And as our modern profit-driven health care systems begin to crumble apart as their dysfunction is revealed, a new way of living will emerge in which people will value financial gain less and will remember that our true nature is to serve one another. You and I can make the world we live in a bit better for ourselves, our friends, and our families by being responsible for our health, making good choices, supporting small local farms, choosing to embrace what life has given to us with gratitude, and pursuing our dreams to create something more.

There is a deep human need to be loved and cared for. Give this gift to yourself because you deserve it.

I wrote this book in honor of you,
in honor of our ancestors who have come before us,
and in honor of our descendants, those who will come after us.

You are not here to suffer. You are here to live, to love, and to heal your suffering. I personally would like to wish you healing, abundance, joy, and good health on your journey.

Ramiel

Product Disclaimer

If you have any systemic medical condition, or are on medications, please consult with a trusted health care provider before trying any of the advice or dietary supplements recommended in this book.

It is impossible for me to know what products or ideas offered in this book may or may not benefit you. I have done my best to provide safe and natural guidelines to support your health and vitality in general. That being said, since every person is unique, it is possible that some of the advice in this book, or products that are recommended, may not suit you.

Furthermore, I have created a business to provide foods and whole food supplements for people who wish to improve their health, Traditional Foods Market, www.traditionalfoods.org. It is important for you to know that I own this business and I have recommended products that I directly profit from.

There is a specific purpose for me to sell products directly. My goal is to give people high quality foods and supplements at a reasonable price. Rather than, for example, simply recommending vitamin C, I have spent the time, energy, and effort to find the highest quality vitamin C on the market, and at the same time, keep the price lower. I truly want to provide superior products that will suit most people, so I share my products with you in the spirit of being helpful and being of service. There is no requirement to buy any products mentioned in the book to be successful with your gum healing.

With that in mind, every product or service you try in this book is done at your own risk and responsibility. The best results for using dietary supplements are obtained by using a method to test whether the supplement is right for you. Some alternative health practitioners provide this service, so do not be afraid to ask for help. At the same time, I know that it can be difficult to find the few good practitioners to help support your health. So do your best to find what works for you. Understand that not everything suggested in this book is exactly right for your particular needs. For example, it is very hard to estimate the dosage and frequency of the products that every unique individual needs to take. And everyone needs changes from day to day and season to season. Nothing in this book is meant to supplant your own inner wisdom or feelings about what is right for you and for what you need to be healthy, but rather, it is to help encourage your connection with it.

Endnotes

Chapter 1

1 Nield-Gehrig, Jill S., and Donald E. Willmann. Introduction. *Foundations of Periodontics for the Dental Hygenist*. Philadelphia: Lippincott Williams & Wilkins, 2003. 131.

2 Genco, Robert J., and Ray C. Williams. *Periodontal Disease and Overall Health: A Clinician's Guide*. Yardley, PA: Professional Audience Communications, 2010. 8. Print.

3 Ibid.

4 "Periodontitis Among Adults Aged ≥30 Years — United States, 2009–2010." *Centers for Disease Control and Prevention*. Centers for Disease Control and Prevention, 22 Nov. 2013. Web. 20 Aug. 2014. http://www.cdc.gov/mmwr/preview/mmwrhtml/su6203a21.htm

5 http://student.ahc.umn.edu/dental/2010/Documents/DentalBioChem/L3-5302-2Apr07.ppt

6 Genco, Robert J., and Ray C. Williams. *Periodontal Disease and Overall Health: A Clinician's Guide*. Yardley, PA: Professional Audience Communications, 2010. Ch. 1. 1. Print.

7 White, Donald J. "Dental Calculus: Recent Insights into Occurrence, Formation, Prevention, Removal and Oral Health Effects of Supragingival and Subgingival Deposits." *European Journal of Oral Sciences* 105.5 (1997): 508-22. Web.

8 Kornman KS. Patients are not equally susceptible to periodontitis: Does this change dental practice and the dental curriculum? *J Dent Educ* 2001;65:777-784.

9 "Types of Gum Disease | Perio.org." *Types of Gum Disease | Perio.org*. N.p., n.d. Web. 22 Aug. 2014. <http://www.perio.org/consumer/types-gum-disease.html>.

10 Darveau RP, Tanner A, Page RC. The microbial challenge in periodontitis. *Periodontol 2000* 1997;14:12-32.

11 Dozens of Authors J. Epidemiology of Periodontal Diseases. J Periodontol 2005;76:1408.

12 Genco, Robert J., and Ray C. Williams. *Periodontal Disease and Overall Health: A Clinician's Guide*. Yardley, PA: Professional Audience Communications, 2010. 8. Print.

13 Genco, Robert J., and Ray C. Williams. *Periodontal Disease and Overall Health: A Clinician's Guide*. Yardley, PA: Professional Audience Communications, 2010. 8. Print.

14 Dozens of Authors J. Epidemiology of Periodontal Diseases. J Periodontol 2005;76:1406-1419.

15 Listgarten MA, Schifter CC, Laster L. 3-year longitudinal study of the periodontal status of an adult population with gingivitis. *J Clin Periodontol* 1985;12:225-238.

16 Ibid.

17 Genco, Robert J., and Ray C. Williams. *Periodontal Disease and Overall Health: A Clinician's Guide*. Yardley, PA: Professional Audience Communications, 2010. 6. Print.

18 "QuickStats: Prevalence of Moderate and Severe Periodontitis* Among Adults Aged 45–74 Years, by Race/Ethnicity and Age Group — National Health and Nutrition Examination Survey, United States, 2009–2010." Centers for Disease Control and Prevention. Centers for Disease Control and Prevention, 18 Jan. 2013. Web. 20 Aug. 2014. <http://www.cdc.gov/mmwr/preview/mmwrhtml/mm6202a6.htm>.

19 Genco, Robert J., and Ray C. Williams. *Periodontal Disease and Overall Health: A Clinician's Guide*. Yardley, PA: Professional Audience Communications, 2010. 12. Print.

20 Ibid. 12.

21 Ibid. 12.

Chapter 2

1 Toverud, Guttorm. *A Survey of the Literature of Dental Caries: Prepared for the Food and Nutrition Board National Research Council*. Washington: National Academy of Sciences, 1952. 127. Print.

2 Masterjohn, Chris. "Understanding Weston Price on Primitive Wisdom — Ancient Doesn't Cut It." *Weston A Price*. N.p., n.d. Web. 17 Sept. 2014. <http://www.westonaprice.org/uncategorized/understanding-weston-price-on-primitive-wisdom-ancient-doesnt-cut-it/>.

3 Fallon, Sally. *The Right Price: Interpreting the Work of Weston Price*. Weston a Price Foundation http://www.westonaprice.org/basicnutrition/right_price.html,

4 Price, W.A. *Nutrition and Physical Degeneration*, 6th Ed. 26.

5 Ibid.

6 Ibid.

7 Ibid., 35.

8 Ibid., 39.

9 Ibid., 27.

10 Price, "Why Dental Caries with Modern Civilizations? V. An Interpretation of Field Studies Previously Reported," 278.

11 op. cit., p. 27.

12 Price, "Why Dental Caries with Modern Civilizations? V. An Interpretation of Field Studies Previously Reported," 278.

13 Ibid., 35.

14 op. cit., p. 38.

15 Ibid., 64.

16 Ibid.

17 Price, *Nutrition and Physical Degeneration*, 6th Ed. 259.

18 Price, "Why Dental Caries with Modern Civilizations? XI. New Light on Loss of Immunity to Some Degenerative Processes Including Dental Caries," 243.

19 Ibid., 244

20 Price, "Why Dental Caries with Modern Civilizations? XI. New Light on Loss of Immunity to Some Degenerative Processes Including Dental Caries," 244.

21 Ibid., 67.

22 Ibid., 68.

23 Ibid., 59.

24 Ibid.

25 Price, "Why Dental Caries with Modern Civilizations? XI. New Light on Loss of Immunity to Some Degenerative Processes Including Dental Caries," 243.

26 Ibid., 244

27 (http://quod.lib.umich.edu/d/dencos/0527912.0077.001/11

78:664?page=root;rgn=main;-size=100;view=image)

28 Price, *Nutrition and Physical Degeneration*, 6th Ed. 260.

29 Pacific Islanders, Diet of, Internet FAQ archives, http://www.faqs.org/nutrition/Ome-Pop/Pacific-Islanders-Diet-of.html

30 "Obesity in the Pacific." *Wikipedia*. Wikimedia Foundation, 24 Aug. 2014. Web. 17 Sept. 2014. <http://en.wikipedia.org/wiki/Obesity_in_the_Pacific>.

31 Price, Weston. "SOME PHASES OF PREVENTIVE DENTISTRY OF SPECIAL CONCERN TO CANADIAN DENTISTS." *Journal of Canadian Dental Society* 1.5 (1935): 199-208. Web.

32 Price, Weston A. *Nutrition and Physical Degeneration*. La Mesa, CA: Price-Pottenger Nutrition Foundation, 2008. Print.

33 Price, W. A. *Nutrition and Physical Degeneration 6th Edition*. La Mesa: Price-Pottenger Nutrition Foundation; 2004: op. cit., p. 441.

34 Ibid., 173.

35 Ibid., 186.

36 Fallon, S. and Enig, M. Australian Aborigines-- Living Off the Fat of the Land, Available At: http://www.westonaprice.org/traditional_diets/australian_aborigines.html

37 op. cit., p. 174.

38 op. cit., p. 171.

39 Price, W. A. *Nutrition and Physical Degeneration 6th Edition*. La Mesa: Price-Pottenger Nutrition Foundation; 2004: op. cit., p. 174.

40 op. cit., p. 275-276.

41 Price, Weston A. *Nutrition and Physical Degeneration*. La Mesa, CA: Price-Pottenger Nutrition Foundation, 2008. Print.

42 Price, Weston A. "Field Studies among Some African Tribes on the Relation of Their Nutrition to the Incidence of Dental Caries and Dental Arch Deformities" *Journal. A.D.A.* 23:888, May 1936.

43 1. SUPPLEMENTARY DATA TABLES, USDA's 1994-96 Continuing Survey of Food Intakes by Individuals, Table Set 12, *US Department of Agriculture, Agricultural Research Service*, http://www.ars.usda.gov/SP2UserFiles/Place/12355000/pdf/Supp.PDF

Chapter 3

1 Hawkins, Harold Fuller. *Applied Nutrition*. La Habra, CA: International College of Applied Nutrition, 1977. 1-12. Print.

2 Ibid.

3 "Alveolar Bone Ppt Presentation." *AuthorSTREAM*. N.p., n.d. Web. 28 Aug. 2014. <http://www.authorstream.com/Presentation/rahul.ahirrao-1764514-alveolar-bone/>.

4 Hawkins, Harold F. "Nutritional Influences on Growth and Development."*International Journal of Orthodontia and Dentistry for Children* 19.3 (1933): 307-12. Web.

5 Hawkins, Harold Fuller. *Applied Nutrition*. La Habra, CA: International College of Applied Nutrition, 1977. 8. Print.12.

6 Ibid., 61.

7 Acharya A1, Kharadi MD, Dhavale R, Deshmukh VL, Sontakke AN. "High Salivary Calcium Level Associated with Periodontal Disease in Indian Subjects--a Pilot Study." Oral Health Prev Dent. 2011;9(2):195-200. (n.d.): n. pag. Web.

8 Ibid. 12-14.

9 Hawkins, Harold Fuller. *Applied Nutrition*. La Habra, CA: International College of Applied Nutrition, 1977. 10-12. Print.

10 Ibid., 12-14.

11 Ibid., 13.

12 "The Pioneers of Nutrition." International Foundation of Nutrition and Health. N.p., n.d. Web. 27 Aug. 2014. <http://www.ifnh.org/Bio%20Page%20.htm>.

13 Page, M. Abrams, L. *Your Body is Your Best Doctor*. New Canaan: Keats Publishing Inc.;1972:196.

14 Forbes, R. *The Hormone Mess And How To Fix It*. 2004: 7.

15 Ibid., 23.

16 Page, Melvin E. *Degeneration, Regeneration*. St. Petersburg, FL: Biochemical Research Foundation, 1949. Page 43. Print.

17 "Central Control of the Autonomic Nervous System and Thermoregulation | Department of Neurobiology and Anatomy - The University of Texas Medical School at Houston. N.p., n.d. Web. 27 Aug. 2014. <http://neuroscience.uth.tmc.edu/s4/chapter03.html>.

18 Page, Melvin E. *Degeneration, Regeneration*. St. Petersburg, FL: Biochemical Research Foundation, 1949. Page 52. Print.

19 Page, Melvin. *Mineral Nutrition*. N.p.: n.p., 1938. 14. Print.

20 Ibid.

21 "Endocrine System." *InnerBody*. N.p., n.d. Web. 27 Aug. 2014. <http://www.innerbody.com/image/endoov.html>.

22 Page, Melvin E., and H. Leon Abrams. *Your Body Is Your Best Doctor!* New Canaan, CT: Keats Pub., 1972. 112-13. Print.

23 Forbes, R. *The Hormone Mess and How to Fix It*. 2004: 12.

24 "One Answer to Cancer." *One Answer to Cancer*. N.p., n.d. Web. 29 Aug. 2014. <http://www.drkelley.com/CANLIVER55.html>.

25 "Researchers Uncover Higher Prevalence of Periodontal Disease in Rheumatoid Arthritis Patients Perio.org." *Researchers Uncover Higher Prevalence of Periodontal Disease in Rheumatoid Arthritis Patients | Perio.org*. N.p., n.d. Web. 29 Aug. 2014. <http://www.perio.org/consumer/arthritis-link>.

26 Page, Melvin E. *Degeneration, Regeneration*. St. Petersburg, FL: Biochemical Research Foundation, 1949. Page 70-71. Print.

27 Ibid., 113-114.

28 Page, Melvin E., and H. Leon. Abrams. *Health vs Disease, a Revolution in Medical Thinking*. St. Petersburg, FL: Page Foundation, 1960. 57. Print.

29 Douard, Veronique, Abbas Asgerally, Yves Sabbagh, Shozo Sugiura, Sue A. Shapses, Donatella Casirola, and Ronaldo P. Ferraris. "Abstract."*National Center for Biotechnology Information*. U.S. National Library of Medicine, 31 July 2005. Web. 29 Aug. 2014. <http://www.ncbi.nlm.nih.gov/pmc/articles/PMC2834550/>.

30 Page, Melvin E., and H. Leon. Abrams. *Health vs Disease, a*

Revolution in Medical Thinking. St. Petersburg, FL: Page Foundation, 1960. 53. Print.

31 2, Chapter. *Profiling Food Consumption in America* (n.d.): n. pag. *USDA*. Web. <http://www.usda.gov/factbook/chapter2.pdf>.

32 Guyenet, Stephan. "Whole Health Source: By 2606, the US Diet Will Be 100 Percent Sugar." *Whole Health Source: By 2606, the US Diet Will Be 100 Percent Sugar*. N.p., n.d. Web. 02 Sept. 2014. <http://wholehealthsource.blogspot.com/2012/02/by-2606-us-diet-will-be-100-percent.html>.

33 Page, Melvin. *Mineral Nutrition.* N.p.: n.p., 1938. 17. Print.

34 "The Dental Cosmos; a Monthly Record of Dental Science. [Vol. 52]." *The Dental Cosmos; a Monthly Record of Dental Science. [Vol. 52]*. N.p., n.d. Web. 28 Aug. 2014. <http://quod.lib.umich.edu/d/decos/0527912.0052.001/1200?q1=gingivitis&node=0527912.0052.001%3A787&view=image&size=125>.

35 "The Journal of the American Dental Association." *The Relationship Between Oral Health and Diabetes Mellitus*. N.p., n.d. Web. 28 Aug. 2014. <http://jada.ada.org/content/139/suppl_5/19S.full>.

36 Rajhans NS, Kohad RM, Chaudhari VG, Mhaske NH. A clinical study of the relationship between diabetes mellitus and periodontal disease. J Indian Soc Periodontol [serial online] 2011 [cited 2014 Aug 29];15:388-92. Available from: http://www.jisponline.com/text.asp?2011/15/4/388/92576

37 Page, Melvin E. *Young Minds with Old Bodies*. Boston: B. Humphries,; Toronto, The Ryerson, 1944. 8. Print.

38 Indirect reference: "Pregnancy gingivitis: History, classification, etiology" Daniel E Ziskin, Gerald J Nesse American journal of orthodontics and oral surgery 1 June 1946 (volume 32 issue 6 Pages A390-A432).

39 "Histology of the Periodontium - Alveolar Process - Bone Remodeling."*Histology of the Periodontium - Alveolar Process - Bone Remodeling*. N.p., n.d. Web. 30 Aug. 2014. <http://www.dental.pitt.edu/informatics/periohistology/en/gu0603.htm>.

40 Mccoy, Gene. "Dental Compression Syndrome: A New Look at an Old Disease." *Journal of Oral Implantology* 25.1 (1999): 35-49. Web

41 Genco, Robert J., and Ray C. Williams. *Periodontal Disease and Overall Health: A Clinician's Guide*. Yardley, PA: Professional Audience Communications, 2010. 6. Print.

42 Moulton, Ruth, Sol Ewen, and William Thieman. "Emotional Factors in Periodontal Disease." Oral Surgery, Oral Medicine, Oral Pathology 5.8 (1952): 833-60. Web.

Chapter 4

1 Hawkins, Harold Fuller. *Applied Nutrition*. La Habra, CA: International College of Applied Nutrition, 1977. 47. Print.

2 "Vitamin A On Trial: Does Vitamin A Cause Osteoporosis?" *Weston A Price*. N.p., n.d. Web. 30 Aug. 2014. <http://www.westonaprice.org/health-topics/abcs-of-nutrition/vitamin-a-on-trial-does-vitamin-a-cause-osteoporosis/>.

3 Hawkins, Harold Fuller. *Applied Nutrition*. La Habra, CA: International College of Applied Nutrition, 1977. 46. Print.

4 "Vitamins in Dental Care." *Vitamins in Dental Care*. N.p., n.d. Web. 30 Aug. 2014. <https://www.seleneriverpress.com/historical-archives/all-archive-articles/115-vitamins-in-dental-care>.

5 Carranza's Clinical Periodontology N.p.: W B Saunders, 2011. Print.

6 "Nutrition Facts." And Analysis for Rice, Brown, Long-grain, Cooked. N.p., n.d. Web. 08 Jan. 2015. <http://nutritiondata.self.com/facts/cereal-grains-and-pasta/5707/2>.

7 "Nutrition Facts." And Analysis for Rice, White, Long-grain, Regular, Cooked. N.p., n.d. Web. 08 Jan. 2015. <http://nutritiondata.self.com/facts/cereal-grains-and-pasta/5712/2>.

8 N. H. Topping and H. F. Fraser. "Mouth Lesions Associated with Dietary Deficiencies in Monkeys." Public Health Reports (1896-1970), Vol. 54, No. 11 (Mar. 17, 1939), pp. 416-431.

9 "Linus Pauling InstituteMicronutrient Research for Optimum Health." *Linus Pauling Institute at Oregon State University*. N.p., n.d. Web. 30 Aug. 2014. <http://lpi.oregonstate.edu/infocenter/vitamins/riboflavin/>.

10 Podolin, Mathew. "Oral Manifestations of the Nutritional Deficiency Diseases." Dental Bytes. N.p., n.d. Web. 30 Aug. 2014. <http://www.dentalbytes.com/dental-treatments/causative-factors-in-dental-caries/oral-manifestations -of-the-nutritional-deficiency-diseases.htm>.

11 "Conservative Nutrition: The Industrial Food Supply and Its Critics, 1915-1985." *EScholarship*. Renner, Martin. Web. 31 Aug. 2014. <http://escholarship.org/uc/item/6nk2s73b>.

12 Toverud, Guttorm. *A Survey of the Literature of Dental Caries*. Washington: n.p., 1952. Pg 472. Print.

13 "Top 10 Foods Highest in Vitamin B5 (Pantothenic Acid)." *Top 10 Foods Highest in Vitamin B5 (Pantothenic Acid)*. N.p., n.d. Web. 31 Aug. 2014. <http://www.healthaliciousness.com/articles/foods-high-in-pantothenic-acid-vitamin-B5.php>.

14 "Top 10 Foods Highest in Vitamin B6." *Top 10 Foods Highest in Vitamin B6*. N.p., n.d. Web. 31 Aug. 2014. <http://www.healthaliciousness.com/articles/foods-high-in-vitamin-B6.php>.

15 "Biotin." Linus Pauling Institute at Oregon State University. N.p., n.d. Web. 22 Oct. 2014. <http://lpi.oregonstate.edu/infocenter/vitamins/biotin/>.

16 "Choline." Linus Pauling Institute at Oregon State University. N.p., n.d. Web. 22 Oct. 2014. <http://lpi.oregonstate.edu/infocenter/othernuts/choline/>.

17 Yu, Yau-Hua, Hsu-Ko Kuo, and Yu-Lin Lai. "The Association Between Serum Folate Levels and Periodontal Disease in Older Adults: Data from the National

Health and Nutrition Examination Survey 2001/02."*Journal of the American Geriatrics Society* 55.1 (2007): 108-13. Web.

18 "Smile-on News." *Association of Chronic Periodontitis and Anaemia*. N.p., n.d. Web. 31 Aug. 2014. <http://www.smile-on-news.com/article/view/association-of-chronic-periodontitis-and-anaemia>.

19 "Severe periodontal destruction in a patient with advanced anemia: A case report" Hatipoglu, Hasan, Mujgan Gungor Hatipoglu, L. Berna Cagirankaya, and Feriha Caglayan. Eur J Dent. Jan 2012; 6(1): 95–100.

20 Landsman, Jonathan. "Vitamin C helps to prevent gum disease." Natural Health 365. Web. 30 Jun 2014. < http://www.naturalhealth365.com/vitamin_c/prevent-gum-disease-1056.html>

21 Pirkko J. Pussinen. "Periodontitis is associated with a low concentration of vitamin C in Plasma." *Clinical and Diagnostic Laboratory Immunology*. 10.5 (2003): 897-902.Web

22 "Conservative Nutrition: The Industrial Food Supply and Its Critics, 1915-1985." *EScholarship*. Renner, Martin. Web. 31 Aug. 2014. <http://escholarship.org/uc/item/6nk2s73b>. Page 130.

23 Podolin, Mathew. "Oral Manifestations of the Nutritional Deficiency Diseases." Dental Bytes. N.p., n.d. Web. 30 Aug. 2014. <http://www.dentalbytes.com/dental-treatments/causative-factors-in-dental-caries/oral-manifestations-of-the-nutritional-deficiency-diseases.htm>.

24 "Vitamins in Dental Care." *Vitamins in Dental Care*. Lee, Royal. Web. 30 Aug. 2014. <https://www.seleneriverpress.com/historical-archives/all-archive-articles/115-vitamins-in-dental-care>.

25 Genco, Robert J., and Ray C. Williams. *Periodontal Disease and Overall Health: A Clinician's Guide*. Yardley, PA: Professional Audience Communications, 2010. 18. Print.

26 Podolin, Mathew. "Oral Manifestations of the Nutritional Deficiency Diseases." Dental Bytes. N.p., n.d. Web. 30 Aug. 2014. <http://www.dentalbytes.com/dental-treatments/causative-factors-in-dental-caries/oral-manifestations-of-the-nutritional-deficiency-diseases.htm>.

27 "A Consideration Of Periodontal Disease." Dental Bytes. Paul H. Belding, D. D. S., AND Leland J. Belding, M. D. Web. <http://www.dentalbytes.com/a-consideration-of-periodontal-disease-post.htm>.

28 "The Effect of Intravenous Vitamin C on the Phosphorus Level Reduction in Hemodialysis Patients: A Double Blind Randomized Clinical Trial." Gholipour Baradari A1, Emami Zeydi A, Espahbodi F, Aarabi M. Web. 31 Aug. 2014. <http://www.ncbi.nlm.nih.gov/pubmed/22634906>.

29 "Vitamin C Supplementation." Vitamin C Overdose/deficiency Symptoms, Benefits, Side Effects. Web. 31 Aug. 2014. <http://www.acu-cell.com/vitc.html#excess>.

30 Lamberton, B.Sc., Rob. "Synthetic Vitamin C : Is It Damaging Your Health?" Nutricula. Web. <http://www.nutriculamagazine.com/synthetic-vitamin-c-is-it-damaging-your-health/>.

31 Mellanby, May. "Periodontal Disease in Dogs (experimental Gingivitis and "pyorrhea")." *The Dental Cosmos* 73.7 (1931): 729-30. Web.

32 Mellanby, Edward. Nutrition and Disease; the Interaction of Clinical and Experimental Work. Edinburgh: Oliver and Boyd, 1934. 28-31. Print.

33 Vitamins in Dental Care." *Vitamins in Dental Care*. Lee, Royal. Web. 30 Aug. 2014. <https://www.seleneriverpress.com/historical-archives/all-archive-articles/115-vitamins- in-dental-care>.

34 Hujoel PP. Vitamin D and Dental Caries: Systematic Review and Meta-analysis. (2012) Nutrition Reviews.

35 "Information on the Latest Vitamin D News and Research." *Vitamin D Council*. Web. 31 Aug. 2014. <https://www.vitamindcouncil.org/health-conditions/periodontal-disease/>.

36 Hawkins, Harold Fuller. *Applied Nutrition*. La Habra, CA: International College of Applied Nutrition, 1977. 61. Print.

37 Masterjohn, Chris. "On the Trail of the Elusive X-Factor: A Sixty-Two-Year-Old Mystery Finally Solved." The Weston A. Price Foundation. 13 Feb. 2008. Web. 16 Aug. 2010. <http://www.westonaprice.org/abcs-of-nutrition/175-x-factor-is-vitamin-k2.html>.

38 Feldman, David, J. Wesley. Pike, and John S. Adams. *Vitamin D*. Amsterdam: Academic, 2011. 997. Print.

39 Mellanby, May. "THE AETIOLOGY OF DENTAL CARIES." *British Medical Journal* (1932): 749-51. Print.

40 There are "30 metabolites of vitamin D" but only the calcitriol, 1.25 $-(OH)_2\ D_3$ of vitamin D3 is active. D2 also has an active metabolite: 1,25- $(OH)_2D_2$ (DeLuca, Hector, F. "History of the discovery of vitamin D and its active metabolites. " BoneKEy Reports (InternationalBone & Mineral Society) 3. 479 (2013): 4. Web. <http://www.nature.com/bonekeyreports/2014/140108/bonekey2013213/full/bonekey2013213.html>

41 Price, Weston. "Control of Dental Caries and Some Associated Degenerative Processes Through Reinforcement of the Diet With Special Activators." *The Journal of the American Dental Association* Vol. XiX. Pages 1339-1369, August. 1932.

42 Wetzel, David. "Cod Liver Oil Manufacturing." The Weston A. Price Foundation. 28 Feb. 2006. Web. 22 Aug. 2010. <http://www.westonaprice.org/cod-liver-oil/183-clo-manufacturing.html>.

43 Fallon, Sally, and Enig, Mary. "Cod Liver Oil Basics and Recommendations." Web.9 Feb 2009, updated 2014. < *http://www.westonaprice.org/health-topics/cod-liver-oil-basics-and-recommendations*>.

44 Fallon, Sally, and Mary Enig. "Cod Liver Oil Basics and Recommendations." The Weston A. Price Foundation. 8 Feb. 2008. Web. 23 Aug. 2010. <http://www.westonaprice.org/cod-liver-oil/238.html#brands>.

45 Møller, Frantz Peckel, and Peter Møller Heyerdahl. Cod-liver Oil and Chemistry. London, Christiania: P. Möller, 1895. Print.

46 Cowan, Thomas S., Sally Fallon, and Jaimen McMillan. The Fourfold Path to Healing: Working with the Laws of Nutrition, Therapeutics, Movement and Meditation in the Art of Medicine. Washington D.C.: NewTrends Pub., 2004. Print.

47 Price, W. A. *Nutrition and Physical Degeneration* 6th Edition. La Mesa: Price-Pottenger Nutrition Foundation; 2004:26.

48 Price, W. A. *Nutrition and Physical Degeneration* 8th Edition. La Mesa: Price-Pottenger Nutrition Foundation; 2008:385.

49 Ibid., 386.

50 Masterjohn, Chris. "On the Trail of the Elusive X-Factor: A Sixty-Two-Year-Old Mystery Finally Solved." Weston A Price. N.p., n.d. Web. 22 Oct. 2014. <http://www.westonaprice.org/health-topics/abcs-of-nutrition/on-the-trail-of-the-elusive-x-factor-a-sixty-two-year-old-mystery-finally-solved/>.

51 Thomson, Ronald Hunter. Naturally Occurring Quinones. London: Acad. Pr., 1971. Print.

52 Ibid.

53 "Top Food Sources of Vitamin K2 (Menaquinone-4)." Top Food Sources of Vitamin K2 (Menaquinone-4). N.p., n.d. Web. 22 Oct. 2014. <http://foodinfo.us/SourcesUnabridged.aspx?Nutr_No=428>. (Note: Also searched for Ethnic foods)

54 Dalby, Matthew. "The Menaquinone (vitamin K2) Content of Animal Products and Fermented Foods." The Call of the Honeyguide. N.p., n.d. Web. 22 Oct. 2014. <http://honey-guide.com/2014/03/10/menaquinones-k2-and-phylloquinone-k1-content-of-animal-products-and-fermented-foods/>.

55 Price, W. A. *Nutrition and Physical Degeneration* 8th Edition. La Mesa: Price-Pottenger Nutrition Foundation; 2008:391.

56 Mercola, Joseph. "Why is Butter Better. Butter Benefits." Web. 07 Dec 2010 <http://articles.mercola.com/sites/articles/archive/2010/12/07/why-is-butter-better.aspx>

57 "Organic Production and Handling Standards." USDA. N.p., n.d. Web. 8 Jan. 2015. <http://www.ams.usda.gov/AMSv1.0/getfile?dDocName=STELDEV3004445>.

58 Podolin, Mathew. "Oral Manifestations of the Nutritional Deficiency Diseases." Dental Bytes. N.p., n.d. Web. 30 Aug. 2014. <http://www.dentalbytes.com/dental-treatments/causative-factors-in-dental-caries/oral-manifestations-of-the-nutritional-deficiency-diseases.htm>.

Chapter 5

1 Wical, Kenneth E., and Charles C. SwDoope. "Studies of Residual Ridge Resorption. Part II. The Relationship of Dietary Calcium and Phosphorus to Residual Ridge Resorption." *The Journal of Prosthetic Dentistry* 32.1 (1974): 13-22. Web.

2 Nishida, Mieko, Sara G. Grossi, Robert G. Dunford, Alex W. Ho, Maurizio Trevisan, and Robert J. Genco. "Calcium and the Risk For Periodontal Disease." Journal of Periodontology 71.7 (2000): 1057-066. Web.

3 Shimazakaki Y et al. "Intake of dairy products and periodontal disease: the Hisayama Study" *Journal of Peridontology*. 79.1 (2008) 131-137. Web.

4 Al-Zahrani, Mohammad S. "Increased Intake of Dairy Products Is Related to Lower Periodontitis Prevalence." *Journal of Periodontology* 77.2 (2006): 289-94. Web.

5 Chatterjee Anirba, Bhattacharya Hirak Dandwal Abhishek. Probiotics in periodontal health and disease. 15. 1 (2011) : 23-28. Web

6 McAfee, Mark. "The Fifteen Things That Pasteurization Kills." *Wise Traditions* Summer (2010): 82. Print.

7 Ibid.

8 The Facts about Real Raw Milk. The WestonA. Price Foundation. <http://www.realmilk.com/ >. Web.

9 Pottenger, Francis. "A Fresh Look at Milk." *Selene River Press*. N.p., n.d. Web. < https://www.seleneriverpress.com/historical-archives/all-archive-articles/194-a-fresh-look-at-milk>.

10 Huggins, Hal A.. *It's All in Your Head: The Link Between Mercury Amalgams and Illness*. 1 ed. New York: Avery Publishing, 1993. Print:155.

11 Mohanty, Rinkee. Nazareth, Nianca. Shirvasta, Neha. "The potential role of probiotics in periodontal health." RSBO. 9.1.(2012) 85-8. Print.

12 Shimazaki, Yoshihiro, Tomoko Shirota, Kazuhiro Uchida, Koji Yonemoto, Yutaka Kiyohara, Mitsuo Iida, Toshiyuki Saito, and Yoshihisa Yamashita. "Intake of Dairy Products and Periodontal Disease: The Hisayama Study." *Journal of Periodontology* 79.1 (2008): 131-37. Web.

13 Page, Melvin E., and H. Leon Abrams. *Your Body Is Your Best Doctor!* New Canaan, CT: Keats Pub., 1972. 129. Print.

14 Page, Melvin E. *Young Minds with Old Bodies*. Boston: B. Humphries,; Toronto, The Ryerson, 1944. 188. Print.

15 Ibid. 113.

16 Young ER. The thyroid gland and the dental practitioner. J Can Dent Assoc. 1989;55:903–7.

17 Fallon, Sally. "The Great Iodine Debate." *Weston A Price*. N.p., n.d. Web. 05 Sept. 2014. <http://www.westonaprice.org/modern-diseases/the-great-iodine-debate/>.

18 Zava, Theodore T., and David T. Zava. "Assessment of Japanese Iodine Intake Based on Seaweed Consumption in Japan: A Literature-based Analysis." *Thyroid Research* 4.1 (2011): 14. Web.

19 Orbak, R., C. Kara, E. Özbek, A. Tezel, and T. Demir. "Effects of Zinc Deficiency on Oral and Periodontal Diseases in Rats." *Journal of Periodontal Research* 42.2 (2007): 138-43. Web.

20 Poleník, P. "Zinc in Etiology of Periodontal Disease." *Medical Hypotheses*40.3 (1993): 182-85. Web.

21 J H Freeland, R J Cousins, and R Schwartz. "Relationship of Mineral Status and Intake to Periodontal Disease." (n.d.): Am

J Clin Nutr July 1976 vol. 29 no. 7 745-749.

22 Warner, Laurie. "Copper-Zinc Imbalance: Unrecognized Consequence of Plant-Based Diets and a Contributor to Chronic Fatigue." *Weston A Price.* N.p., n.d. Web. 05 Sept. 2014. <http://www.westonaprice.org/modern-diseases/copper-zinc-imbalance-unrecognized-consequence-of-plant-based-diets-and-a-contributor-to-chronic-fatigue/>.

23 Colagar, Abasalt Hosseinzadeh, Eisa Tahmasbpour Marzony, and Mohammad Javad Chaichi. "Zinc Levels in Seminal Plasma Are Associated with Sperm Quality in Fertile and Infertile Men." *Nutrition Research* 29.2 (2009): 82-88. Web.

24 "Linus Pauling InstituteMicronutrient Research for Optimum Health." Linus Pauling Institute at Oregon State University. N.p., n.d. Web. 06 Sept. 2014. <http://lpi.oregonstate.edu/infocenter/minerals/magnesium/>.

25 Fallon, Sally. "The Salt of the Earth." *Weston A Price.* N.p., n.d. Web. 05 Sept. 2014. <http://www.westonaprice.org/health-topics/abcs-of-nutrition/the-salt-of-the-earth/>.

26 Satin, Morton. "Salt and Our Health." *Weston A Price.* N.p., n.d. Web. 05 Sept. 2014. <http://www.westonaprice.org/health-topics/abcs-of-nutrition/salt-and-our-health/>.

27 Genco, Robert J., and Ray C. Williams. *Periodontal Disease and Overall Health: A Clinician's Guide.* Yardley, PA: Professional Audience Communications, 2010. 256. Print.

28 Peat, Ray. "Diabetes, Scleroderma, Oils and Hormones." *Diabetes, Scleroderma, Oils and Hormones.* N.p., n.d. Web. 05 Sept. 2014. <http://raypeat.com/articles/articles/diabetes.shtml>.

Chapter 6

1 Price, W. A. *Nutrition and Physical Degeneration 6th Edition.* La Mesa: Price-Pottenger Nutrition Foundation; 2004: Chapter 10.

2 William. "PROLIFIC SOURCES OF PYORRHEA." (n.d.): n. pag. Web. <http://www.dentalbytes.com/health-education/a-cyst-in-no-mans-land/prolific-sources-of-pyorrhea.htm>.

3 Wedman, Betty. "Letters, Spring 2013." Weston A Price. N.p., n.d. Web. 17 Nov. 2014. <http://www.westonaprice.org/uncategorized/letters-spring-2013/>.

4 Iron absorption in man: ascrobic acid and dose-depended inhibition. *American Journal of Clinical Nutrition.* Jan 1989. 49(1):140-144.

5 Davidson, Lena. "Iron Bioavailablity from Weaning Foods: The Effect of Phytic Acid" Macronutrient Interactions: Impact on Child Health and Nutrition by US Agency for International Development Food and Agricultural Organization of the United Nations. 1996:22.

6 Tannenbaum and others. *Vitamins and Minerals in Food Chemistry*, 2nd edition. OR Fennema, ed. Marcel Dekker, Inc., New York, 1985, p 445.

7 Ibid.

8 Singh M and Krikorian D. Inhibition of trypsin activity in vitro by phytate. *Journal of Agricultural and Food Chemistry* 1982 30(4):799-800.

9 Ibid.

10 "Fermented cereals a global perspective. Table of contents.." *FAO: FAO Home.* N.p., n.d. Web. 13 Sept. 2010. <http://www.fao.org/docrep/x2184E/x2184E00.htm >

11 Monastyrsky, Konstantin. "Investigative Report: Why Supplements Got Bad Rap?" GutSense.org. N.p., n.d. Web. 30 Dec. 2014. <http://www.gutsense.org/reports/myth.html>.

12 Barnett Cohen and Lafayette B. Mendel. Experimental Scurvy of the Guinea Pig in Relation to The Diet, *J. Biol. Chem.* 1918 35: 425-453.

13 Barnett Cohen and Lafayette B. Mendel. Experimental Scurvy of the Guinea Pig in Relation to The Diet, *J. Biol. Chem.* 1918 35: 425-453.

14 Nagel, Ramiel. *Cure Tooth Decay: Remineralize Cavities and Repair Your Teeth Naturally.* Los Gatos, CA: Golden Child Publishing; 2011: 63

15 Hess, Alfred F. *Scurvy, past and present.* Philadelphia: J.B. Lippincott Company (1920):111

16 McKenzie-Parnell JM and Davies NT. Destruction of Phytic Acid During Home Breadmaking.*Food Chemistry* 1986 22:181–192.

17 As Dr. Kaayla Daniel reports in *The Whole Soy Story: The Dark Side of America's Favorite Health Food*

18 Ibid., 41.

19 Daniel, Kaayla. "The Little Known Soy-Gluten Connection." Weston A Price. N.p., n.d. Web. 17 Nov. 2014.

20 Mellanby, Edward J. The Rickets-Producing and Anti-Calcifying Action of Phytate *J.Physiol.* (1949) 109, 488-533 547.593:612.751.1

21 CCVIII. PHYTIC ACID AND THE RICKETSPRODUCING ACTION OF CEREALS BY DOUGLAS CREESE HARRISON AD EDWARD MELLANBY From the Field Laboratory, University of Sheffield, and the Department of Biochemistry, Queen's University, Belfast (Received 11 August 1939)

22 Mellanby Edward. "The Rickets-producing and anti-calcifying action of phytate. "*Journal of Physiology.* 109 (1949) :488-533. Print

23 Khadilkar AV. "Vitamin D deficiency in Indian Adolescents." *Indian Paediatrics.* 47 (2010); 756-757. Print

24 Rubel, William. "William Rubel on Bread Ovens in the French Alps." *Rachel Laudan.* N.p., n.d. Web. 13 Sept. 2014. <http://www.rachellaudan.com/2009/03/william-rubel-on-bread-ovens-in-the-french-alps.html>.

25 "Nutrition Facts." *And Analysis for Rice, White, Long-grain, Regular, Cooked.* N.p., n.d. Web. 08 Sept. 2014. <http://nutritiondata.self.com/facts/cereal-grains-and-pasta/5712/2>.

26 Ologhobo AD and Fetuga BL. Distribution of Phosphorus and Phytate in Some Nigerian Varieties of Legumes and some Effects of Processing. *Journal of Food Science* 1984 Volume 49.

27 Unpublished interview with Grandmother from Outer Hebrides.

28 Macfarlane, Bezwoda, Bothwell, Baynes, Bothwell, MacPhail, Lamparelli, Mayet. "inhibitory effect of nuts on iron absorption." *The American Journal of Clinical Nutrition* 47 (1988): 270-274. Print.

29 Ibid.

30 Ibid.

31 N. R. Reddy, Shridhar K. Sathe. *Food Phytates.* 1 ed. Boca Raton, FL: CRC Press, 2001. Print.

32 McGlone, John, and Wilson G. Pond. *Pig Production: Biological Principles and Applications.* 1 ed. Albany: Delmar Cengage Learning, 2002. Print.

33 Trinidad, Trinidad P, Mallillin Aida C, Valdez Divinagracia H. "Dietary fiber from coconut flour: A functional food." *Innovative Food Science and Emerging Technologies.* 7.4 (2006) 309-317

34 Milne Bavid B. Nielsen Forrest H. "The interaction between dietary fructose and magnesium adversely affects macro-mineral homeostasis in men." *Journal of the American College of Nutrition.* 19.1. (2000) 31-37.

35 Ivature R. Kies C. "Mineral balances in humans as affected by fructose, high fructose corn syrup and sucrose. " *Plant foods for Human Nutrition* 42. (1992) 143-151.

36 Huggins, Hal A.. *It's All in Your Head: The Link Between Mercury Amalgams and Illness.* 1 ed. New York: Avery Publishing, 1993. Print:156.

37 Heaney, Anthony. "UCLA's Jonsson Comprehensive Cancer Center : In the News : Pancreatic Cancers Use Fructose, Common in a Western Diet, to Fuel Growth." UCLA's Jonsson Comprehensive Cancer Center : Cancer Treatment and Research. 3 Aug. 2010. Web. 01 Sept. 2010. <http://www.cancer.ucla.edu/Index.aspx?page=644&recordid=385&returnURL=/index.aspx>.

38 "Fructooligosaccharide." Wikipedia. Wikimedia Foundation, 18 Nov. 2014. Web. 19 Nov. 2014. <http://en.wikipedia.org/wiki/Fructooligosaccharide>.

39 Burt, Brian A. "The use of sorbitol- and xylitol-sweetened chewing gum in caries control." *Journal of the American Dental Association* Vol 137, No 2, 190–196. Jan. 2008 <http://jada.ada.org/cgi/content/abstract/137/2/190>.

40 Nagel, Ramiel. "Agave Nectar, the High-Fructose Health Food Fraud (May 2009) Townsend Letter for Doctors & Patients." N.p., n.d. Web. 19 Nov. 2014. <http://www.townsendletter.com/May2009/agave0509.html>.

41 Bournay L. Casanave D, Delfort b. Hillion G. Chorde J.A. "New heterogeneous process for biodiesel production: A way to improve the quality and the value of the crude glycerin produced by biodiesel plants." Catalysis Today. 106.104 (2005): 190-192

42 Nagel, Ramiel. *Cure Tooth Decay: Remineralize Cavities and Repair Your Teeth Naturally.* Los Gatos, CA: Golden Child Publishing; 2011: 57. Print.

43 Ibid.

44 Nagel, Ramiel Cure Tooth Decay: Remineralize Cavities and Repair Your Teeth Naturally. Los Gatos, CA: Golden Child Publishing; 2011: 57. Print.

45 Nagel, Ramiel. *Cure Tooth Decay: Remineralize Cavities and Repair Your Teeth Naturally.* Los Gatos, CA: Golden Child Publishing; 2011: 56-58

46 Foster, Karen. "There Are Shocking Differences Between Raw Honey And The Processed Golden Honey Found In Grocery Retailers." Web. 31 Dec. 2014. <http://preventdisease.com/news/13/071913_Shocking-Difference-Between-Raw-Honey-And-The-Processed-Golden-Honey-Found-In-Grocery-Retailers.shtml>.

47 Olmstead, Larry. "Goodbye Fancy, So Long Grade B: Making Sense Of Maple Syrup." Forbes. Forbes Magazine, n.d. Web. 14 Jan. 2015. <http://www.forbes.com/sites/larryolmsted/2014/04/02/goodbye-fancy-so-long-grade-b-making-sense-of-maple-syrup/>.

48 APEDA. "Jaggery and Confectionary." Ministry of Commerce and Industry. Government of India. Web. <http://www.apeda.gov.in/apedawebsite/SubHead_Products/Jaggery_and_Confectionary.htm>

49 Nagel, Ramiel. *Cure Tooth Decay: Remineralize Cavities and Repair Your Teeth Naturally.* Los Gatos, CA: Golden Child Publishing; 2011: 55. Print.

50 Fallon, S. *Nourishing Traditions.* Washington, DC: New Trends; 1999:13-14.

51 Fallon, Sally. "Trans Fats in the Food Supply." Weston A Price. N.p., n.d. Web. 19 Nov. 2014. <http://www.westonaprice.org/health-topics/trans-fats-in-the-food-supply/>.

52 Federal Register, 1985.

53 Fallon, Sally, and Mary Enig. "The Great Con-ola." The Weston A. Price Foundation. 28 July 2002. Web. 01 Sept. 2010. <http://www.westonaprice.org/know-your-fats/559-the-great-con-ola.html>.

54 Enig, Mary, and Sally Fallon. "The Skinny on Fats." The Weston A. Price Foundation. 01 Sept. 2001. Web. 02 Sept. 2010. <http://www.westonaprice.org/know-your-fats/526-skinny-on-fats.html>.

55 Peat, Ray. "Diabetes, Scleroderma, Oils and Hormones." *Diabetes, Scleroderma, Oils and Hormones.* N.p., n.d. Web. 08 Sept. 2014. <http://raypeat.com/articles/articles/diabetes.shtml>.

56 Errico, Sally. "Olive Oil's Dark Side." N.p., n.d. Web. 31 Dec. 2014. <http://www.newyorker.com/books/page-turner/olive-oils-dark-side>.

57 Davidson, Lena. "Iron Bioavailablity from Weaning Foods: The Effect of Phytic Acid" Macronutrient Interactions: Impact on Child Health and Nutrition by US Agency for International Development Food and Agricultural Organization of the United Nations. 1996:23.

58 "Soy Alert!" The Weston A. Price Foundation. Web. 02 Sept. 2010. <http://www.westonaprice.org/soy-alert.html>.

59 Page, Melvin E., and H. Leon Abrams. *Your Body Is Your Best Doctor!* New Canaan, CT: Keats Pub., 1972. 136. Print.

60 Hansen, Richard. "GOOD TEETH FOR GOOD HEALTH." *GOOD TEETH FOR GOOD HEALTH*. N.p., n.d. Web. 08 Sept. 2014. <http://lightparty.com/Health/Teeth-GoodHealth.html>.

61 "Ardent Light - The Link Between B12 Deficiency & Coffee." *Ardent Light*. N.p., n.d. Web. 08 Sept. 2014. <http://www.ardentlight.com/help/b12.php>.

62 Page, Melvin E., and H. Leon Abrams. *Your Body Is Your Best Doctor!* New Canaan, CT: Keats Pub., 1972. 137. Print.

63 Albandar, Jasim M., Charles F. Streckfus, Margo R. Adesanya, and Deborah M. Winn. "Cigar, Pipe, and Cigarette Smoking as Risk Factors for Periodontal Disease and Tooth Loss." *Journal of Periodontology* 71.12 (2000): 1874-881. Web.

64 Beddoe, Dr. A.F. "Chapter 4." *Theory of Biological Ionization as Applied to Human Nutrition*. N.p.: Advanced Ideals Institute, n.d. 33. Print.

65 Page, Melvin E., and H. Leon Abrams. *Your Body Is Your Best Doctor!* New Canaan, CT: Keats Pub., 1972. 141-142. Print.

66 Fallon, Sally. "The Salt of the Earth." Weston A Price. N.p., n.d. Web. 19 Nov. 2014. <http://www.westonaprice.org/health-topics/abcs-of-nutrition/the-salt-of-the-earth/>.

67 Hawkins, Harold Fuller. *Applied Nutrition*. La Habra, CA: International College of Applied Nutrition, 1977. 145-146, Print.

68 Ibid., 51.

69 Mullally, Brian H., Wilson A. Coulter, Julia D. Hutchinson, and Heather A. Clarke. "Current Oral Contraceptive Status and Periodontitis in Young Adults." *Journal of Periodontology* 78.6 (2007): 1031-036. Web.

70 "Fluoride Action Network." *Fluoride Action Network*. N.p., n.d. Web. 10 Sept. 2014.

71 "FLUORIDE FREE WATER." *: Fluoride Exposure: A Major Risk Factor in Periodontal Disease Which Contributes to Progression of Diabetes, Cardiovascular Disease and Risk of Premature Birth*. N.p., n.d. Web. 10 Sept. 2014.

72 Genco, Robert J., and Ray C. Williams. "Chapter 2." *Periodontal Disease and Overall Health: A Clinician's Guide*. Yardley, PA: Professional Audience Communications, 2010. N. pag. Print.

73 Bavarian State Ministry Of Education And Cultural Affairs, 80327 Munich.*Bavarian State Ministry of Education and Cultural Affairs* (n.d.): n. pag. <http://www.magdahavas.com/wordpress/wp-content/uploads/2010/09/German_Swiss_Wifi_In-Schools_Warn.pdf>

74 Tilden, J. H. *Impaired Health; Its Cause and Cure; a Repudiation of the Conventional Treatment of Disease*. Denver, Col.: J.H. Tilden, 1917. Print.

75 Shelton, Herbert M. Orthotrophy. San Antonio, TX: Dr. Shelton's Health School, 1969. Print. < http://drbass.com/orthopathy/chapter9.html>

76 "Mercury From Amalgam Fillings:." *Mercury From Amalgam Fillings:*. N.p., n.d. Web. 13 Sept. 2014. <http://www.flcv.com/periodon.html>.

77 Lichtenberg H, "Symptoms before and after proper amalgam removal in relation to serum-globulin reaction to metals", Journal of Orthomolecular Medicine,1996, 11(4): 195-203. <http://orthomolecular.org/library/jom/1993/pdf/1993-v08n03-p145.pdf>

78 Ibid.

79 Ibid.

80 Galvanic Currents. <http://www.mercuryexposure.info/science/galvanic-reactions/item/559-dr-rich-chanin-dmd-discusses-galvanic-currents-and-dental-mercury-amalgam-silver-fillings>.

81 "Mercury From Amalgam Fillings:." *Mercury From Amalgam Fillings:*. N.p., n.d. Web. 13 Sept. 2014. <http://www.flcv.com/periodon.html>.

82 Mutter, J. Curth, A. Naumann, J. Deth, R. "Does inorganic mercury play a role in Alzheimer's disease? A systematic review and an integrated molecular mechanism." Journal of Alzheimer's Disease. 22.2 (2010) : 357-74 Print

83 Breiner, Mark A. Whole-body Dentistry: A Complete Guide to Understanding the Impact of Dentistry on Total Health. Fairfield, CT: Quantum Health, 2011. Print.

84 Knight, Galen, and Kaayla Daniel. N.p., n.d. Web. < http://www.westonaprice.org/health-topics/mad-as-a-hatter/ >.

85 "Calcium/Phosphorus Strategy." *Calcium/Phosphorus Strategy*. N.p., n.d. Web. 13 Sept. 2014. <http://www.beatcfsandfms.org/html/CalciumPhosphate.html>.

86 Adams, Mike. "Why Flu Shots Are the Greatest Medical Fraud in History." NaturalNews. N.p., n.d. Web. 31 Dec. 2014. <http://www.naturalnews.com/047942_flu_shots_medical_fraud_vaccine_quackery.html>.

87 Cdc/ncird. Vaccine Excipient & Media Summary - Excipients Included in U.S. Vaccines, by Vaccine - Modified Jan 2014 (n.d.): n. pag. Centers for Disease Control and Prevention. Web. <http://www.cdc.gov/vaccines/pubs/pinkbook/downloads/appendices/b/excipient-table-2.pdf>.

Chapter 7

1 "Ayurveda and the Treatment of Digestive Disease | CA College of Ayurveda." *Ayurveda and the Treatment of Digestive Disease | CA College of Ayurveda*. N.p., n.d. Web. 13 Sept. 2014. <http://www.ayurvedacollege.com/articles/drhalpern/clinical/digestive>.

2 Mishra, Vaidya. "Vaidya Mishra's Shaka Vansya Ayurveda." Shaka Vansya Ayurveda. N.p., n.d. Web. 05 Jan. 2011. <http://www.vaidyamishra.com/>.

3 Gunter, John. "Nutritional Aspect of Dental Disease." *Nutritional Aspect of Dental Disease*. N.p., n.d. Web. 16 Sept. 2014. <https://seleneriverpress.com/historical-archives/all-archive-articles/282-nutritional-aspect-of-dental-disease>.

4 General idea inspired by RBTI (Reams Biological Theory of Ionization).

5 "Digestive Enzyme." Wikipedia. Wikimedia Foundation, 19 Nov.

2014. Web. 24 Nov. 2014.

6 Waters, John. "Correctable Systemic Disorders Indicated by Presence of Salivary Calculus." N.p., n.d. Web. <https://www.seleneriverpress.com/historical-archives-old/all-archive-articles/166-correctable-systemic-disorders-indicated-by-presence-of-salivary-calculus>.

7 Title: Review of Current Dental Literature; Pyorrhea Alveolaris [Volume 53, Issue: 3, March, 1911, pp. 375-376]. http://quod.lib.umich.edu/d/dencos/0527912.0053.001/399>.

8 Richards, Byron J. "Cleaning the Lymph system." Wellness Resources. Web. < http://www.wellnessresources.com/health_topics/detoxification/lymph.php>

9 Mehl-Madrona, Lewis. "Sweat Lodge." *The Journal of Alternative and Complementary Medicine.* (June 2010): 609-610. Print.

10 Krop, J. "Chemical Sensitivity After Intoxication at Work with Solvents: Response to Sauna Therapy." *The Journal of Alternative and Complementary Medicine.* 4.1 (Spring 1998): 77-86. Print.

11 "The Milk Cure: Real Milk Cures Many Diseases - A Campaign for Real..." A Campaign for Real Milk. N.p., n.d. Web. 24 Nov. 2014. <http://www.realmilk.com/health/milk-cure/>.

12 Gala, Dhiren, D. R. Gala, and Sanjay Gala. *Juice-Diet for Perfect Health.*

13 Daniel, Kaayla. "The Surprising, All-Natural Anti Nutrients and Toxins in Plant Food." Weston A. Price Foundation. Web. 29 Mar 2010. < The Surprising, All-Natural Anti-Nutrients and Toxins in Plant Foods>

14 Nagel, Ramiel. *Cure Tooth Decay: Remineralize Cavities and Repair Your Teeth Naturally.* Los Gatos, CA: Golden Child Publishing; 2011: 61

15 Pirtle, Kathryne. "Acid Reflux: A Red Flag. A Precursor to Chronic Illness." The Weston A. Price Foundation. 25 Jun 2010.Web. < http://www.westonaprice.org/modern-diseases/acid-reflux-a-red-flag/>

16 Van het Hof, Karin H. West, Clive. Weststrate, Jan and Hautvast Joseph. "Dietary Factors That Affect the Bioavailability of Carotenoids." *Journal of Nutrition.* 130.3 (2000): 503-506.

17 Vonderplanitz, Aajonus. *The Recipe for Living without Disease.* Santa Monica: Carnelian Bay Castle, 2002. 47-56. Print.

18 Ibid.

Chapter 8

1 Dickson, Charles. Health Benefits of Kelp. Mother Earth News. August/Sept 1999. Web. < http://www.motherearthnews.com/natural-health/health-benefits-kelp-zmaz99aszsto.aspx#axzz3MaFzOPk5>

2 The Big Fat Surprise <http://www.thebigfatsurprise.com/>

3 "Fats and Cholesterol: Out with the Bad, In with the Good." The Nutrition Source. N.p., n.d. Web. 03 Oct. 2014. <http://www.hsph.harvard.edu/nutritionsource/fats-full-story/>.

4 Hawkins, Harold Fuller. Applied Nutrition. La Habra, CA: International College of Applied Nutrition, 1977. 145-146, Print.

5 Nagel, Ramiel. *Cure Tooth Decay: Remineralize Cavities and Repair Your Teeth Naturally.* Los Gatos, CA: Golden Child Publishing; 2011: 58.

6 Hahn, Sandrine. "To Barbecue or Not to Barbecue?" N.p., n.d. Web. <https://nourishingourselves.wordpress.com/2012/05/27/to-barbecue-or-not-to-barbecue/>.

7 Pottenger, F. M. "Hydrophilic Colloidal Diet." American Journal of Digestive Diseases 5.2 (1938): 96-99. Web.

8 Nagel, Ramiel. *Cure Tooth Decay: Remineralize Cavities and Repair Your Teeth Naturally.* Los Gatos, CA: Golden Child Publishing; 2011: 58. Print.

9 Andrews, Ryan. "Forget Calorie Counting: Try This Calorie Control Guide for Men and Women." Precision Nutrition. N.p., n.d. Web. 05 Oct. 2014. <http://www.precisionnutrition.com/calorie-control-guide>.

10 Taubes, Gary. *Why We Get Fat.* New York: Anchor Books. 2011. Print.

11 Stone, Matt. "Paleo Fail - 180 Degree Health." 180 Degree Health. N.p., n.d. Web. 04 Oct. 2014. <http://180degreehealth.com/paleo-fail/>.

12 Pierre, Brian. "Carb Controversy: Why Low-carb Diets Have Got It All Wrong." Precision Nutrition. N.p., n.d. Web. 04 Oct. 2014. <http://www.precisionnutrition.com/low-carb-diets>.

13 Gary Taubes, The Aktins Diet, to name two.

14 Monastyrsky, Konstantin. "The Ingredients of Longevity Nutrition." GutSense.org. N.p., n.d. Web. 15 Dec. 2014. <http://www.gutsense.org/gutsense/nutrition.html>.

15 Otuechere CA, et al., 2013. Virgin coconut oil protects against liver damage in albino rats challenged with the anti-folate combination, trimethoprim-sulfamethoxazole. J Basic Clin Physiol Pharmacol. 28:1-5.

16 Brownstein, David. *Salt Your Way to Health.* 2nd ed. Broomfield Hills, MI: Medical Alternative Press. 2006. Print.

17 "Studies Show Eating Factory Farmed Animal Products Leads to Heart Disease and Cancer." Factory Farm Facts. N.p., n.d. Web. 2 Jan. 2015. <http://www.factoryfarmfacts.com/2012/05/28/studies-show-eating-factory-farmed-animal-products-causes-heart-disease-and-cancer/>.

18 Mastering Nutrition with the Symptom Survey: The Manual for Balancing Body Chemistry with Whole Foods and Herbs. San Diego: IFNH, 2003. 146-47. Print. Can be see also at: < http://www.curetoothdecay.com/Dentistry/melvin_page_dentist.htm>

19 Appleton, Nancy, and G. N. Jacobs. Stopping Inflammation: Relieving the Cause of Degenerative Diseases. Garden City Park, NY: Square One, 2005. 132-35. Print.

20 Heard, George W. "Chapter 17." *Man versus Toothache.* Milwaukee: Lee Foundation for Nutritional Research, 1952. Print.

21 Heard, George W. *Man versus Toothache.* Milwaukee: Lee Foundation for Nutritional Research, 1952. Print.

Chapter 9

1 Memon, Anjum, Sara Godward, Dillwyn Williams, Iqbal Siddique, and Khalid Al-Saleh. "Dental X-rays and the Risk of Thyroid Cancer: A Case-control Study." Acta Oncologica 49.4 (2010): 447-53. Web.

2 Neuberger JS, Brownson RC, Morantz RA, Chin TD. "Association of Brain Cancer with Dental X-rays and Occupation in Missouri." Cancer Detection and Prevention [1991, 15(1):31-34].

3 Ecenbarger, William. "How Dentists Rip Us Off." Readers Digest 10 Mar. 1997: n. pag. Web.

4 Wible, Pamela. "What I've Learned from Saving Physicians from Suicide." KevinMD.com. N.p., 27 May 2013. Web. 20 Jan. 2015. <http://www.kevinmd.com/blog/2013/05/learned-saving-physicians-suicide.html>.

5 "Dental Student Debt." Dental Student Debt. N.p., n.d. Web. 14 Oct. 2014. <http://www.asdanet.org/debt.aspx>.

6 Hefti, A. F. "Periodontal Probing." *Critical Reviews in Oral Biology & Medicine* 8.3 (1997): 336-56. Web.

7 "WHAT IS A PERIODONTIST?" Web. <http://www.perio.org/consumer/periodontist2.htm>.

8 Nield-Gehrig, Jill S., and Donald E. Willmann. Foundations of Periodontics for the Dental Hygenist. Philadelphia: Lippincott Williams & Wilkins, 2003. 257. Print.

9 Ibid.

10 Phillips, Joseph E. Acquiring and Maintaining Oral Health: Through the Blotting Procedure and Total Mouth Hygiene. Osseo, WI: PHB, 1972. 10. Print. Available at www.toothwizards.com

11 Ibid.

12 Ibid., 258.

13 Alves, Renato V., Luciana Machion, Marcio Z. Casati, Francisco H. Nociti, Antonio W. Sallum, and Enilson A. Sallum. "Attachment Loss after Scaling and Root Planing with Different Instruments. A Clinical Study." Journal of Clinical Periodontology 31.1 (2004): 12-15. Web.

14 Friedman, Jay W. The Intelligent Consumer's Complete Guide to Dental Health: How to Maintain Your Dental Health and Avoid Being Overcharged and Overtreated. Bloomington, IN: 1st Library, 2002. Print. 97.

15 Ibid., 98.

16 Ibid., 102.

17 Ibid., 104.

18 Ibid., 108.

19 "Treatments | Perio.org." Treatments | Perio.org. N.p., n.d. Web. 17 Oct. 2014. <http://www.perio.org/consumer/procedures.htm>.

20 Scannapieco, Frank A. Treatment of Periodontal Disease. Philadelphia, PA: W.B. Saunders, 2010. 1. Print.

21 Ibid.

22 Nield-Gehrig, Jill S., and Donald E. Willmann. Foundations of Periodontics for the Dental Hygenist. Philadelphia: Lippincott Williams & Wilkins, 2003. 256. Print.

23 Discussion with a dentist specializing in alternative gum disease treatments.

24 This study is currently unpublished, and can be read at curegumdisease.com

25 Currently Unpublished, may be published in Dent. J. 2014, 2, 1-x; doi:10.3390/dj20x000x by the time this book is released.

26 Harrel, Stephen K., Thomas G. Wilson, and Francisco Rivera-Hidalgo. "A Videoscope for Use in Minimally Invasive Periodontal Surgery." Journal of Clinical Periodontology 40.9 (2013): 868-74. Web.

27 Scannapieco, Frank A. Treatment of Periodontal Disease. Philadelphia, PA: W.B. Saunders, 2010. Print. 1.

28 Isidor, Flemming, and Thorkild Karring. "Long-term Effect of Surgical and Non-surgical Periodontal Treatment. A 5-year Clinical Study." Journal of Periodontal Research 21.5 (1986): 462-72. Web.

29 Heitz-Mayfield, L. J. A., L. Trombelli, F. Heitz, I. Needleman, and D. Moles. "A Systematic Review of the Effect of Surgical Debridement vs. Non-surgical Debridement for the Treatment of Chronic Periodontitis." Journal of Clinical Periodontology 29.S3 (2002): 92-102. Web.

30 Scannapieco, Frank A. Treatment of Periodontal Disease. Philadelphia, PA: W.B. Saunders, 2010. 39. Print. 68.

31 Ibid., 84.

32 Ibid., 106.

33 Pulsed Nd:YAG Laser Treatment for Failing Dental Implants Due to Peri-implantitis. Web. <http://www.lanap.com/pdf/SPIE_LAPIP_abstract_March_2014_8929-16.pdf>.

34 Scannapieco, Frank A. Treatment of Periodontal Disease. Philadelphia, PA: W.B. Saunders, 2010. 39. Print. 119.

35 Sgolastra F, Petrucci A, Severino M, Gatto R, Monaco A.,"Periodontitis, implant loss and peri-implantitis. A meta-analysis.." Clin Oral Implants Res 2013 Dec 31. doi: 10.1111/clr.12319. (2013).

36 Cook, Douglas DDS "Rescued by My Dentist.": 125.

37 Jones, Marilyn. "Titanium Dental Implants Pose Serious Health Risks to the Allergy Sensitive - Dr. Marilyn K Jones." Dr Marilyn K Jones. N.p., 05 Nov. 2013. Web. 17 Dec. 2014. <http://www.marilynkjonesdds.com/1432/titanium-dental-implants-pose-serious-health-risks-allergy-sensitive/>.

38 Munro-Hall, Graeme. Toxic Dentistry Exposed. 66-67. Print.

39 Ibid.

40 Rahul Bhola, Shaily M. Bhola, Corrosion in Titanium Dental Implants/Prostheses - A Review. Trends Biomater. Artif. Organs, 25(1), 34-46 (2011). Available at: <http://medind.nic.in/taa/t11/i1sji/taat11i1sjip34.pdf>

41 "Galvanic Corrosion." Wikipedia. Wikimedia Foundation, n.d. Web. 18 Dec. 2014. <http://en.wikipedia.org/wiki/Galvanic_corrosion>.

42 Munro-Hall, Graeme. Toxic Dentistry Exposed. 66-67. Print.

43 Baylin, Michael. "Dental Implants: An Integrative Perspective." Weston A Price. N.p., n.d. Web. 17 Oct. 2014. <http://www.westonaprice.org/holistic-healthcare/dental-implants-an-integrative-perspective/>.

44 Scannapieco, Frank A. Treatment of Periodontal Disease. Philadelphia, PA: W.B. Saunders, 2010. 35-39. Print.

45 Ibid.

46 Ibid.

47 Uttamani, Juhi, Imaad Shaikh, and Varun Kulkarni. "Use of Lasers in Nonsurgical Periodontal Therapy." Ed. Rajiv Saini. International Journal of Experimental Dental Science 2 (2013): 29-32. Web.

48 Ibid.

49 Ibid.

50 Nevins ML(1), Camelo M, Schupbach P, Kim SW, Kim DM, Nevins M. Human clinical and histologic evaluation of laser-assisted new attachment procedure. Int J Periodontics Restorative Dent. 2012 Oct;32(5):497-507.

51 Liu, Cheing-Meei, Lein-Tuan Hou, Man-Ying Wong, and Wan–Hong Lan. "Comparison of Nd:YAG Laser Versus Scaling and Root Planing in Periodontal Therapy." Journal of Periodontology 70.11 (1999): 1276-282. Web.

52 Uttamani, Juhi, Imaad Shaikh, and Varun Kulkarni. "Use of Lasers in Nonsurgical Periodontal Therapy." Ed. Rajiv Saini. International Journal of Experimental Dental Science 2 (2013): 29-32. Web.

53 Reza Birang, Parichehr Behfarnia, et al. Evaluation of the Effects of Nd:YAG Laser Compared to Scaling and Root Planing Alone on Clinical Periodontal Parameters. J Periodontol Implant Dent 2010; 1(2): 25-28 http://dentistry.tbzmed.ac.ir/jpid/index.php/jpid/article/viewFile/29/15.

54 Nevins M, Kim SW, Camelo M, and Martin IS. "A Prospective 9-month Human Clinical Evaluation of Laser-Assisted New Attachment Procedure (LANAP) Therapy." Int J Periodontics Restorative Dent. 2014 Jan-Feb;34(1):21-7. doi: 10.11607/prd.1848.

55 Carroll, Judy. "The Cost of Periodontal Disease (Gum Disease) Treatments." N.p., n.d. Web. <http://periopeak.com/blog/the-cost-of-periodontal-disease-treatments/>.

56 Phillips, Joseph E. Acquiring and Maintaining Oral Health: Through the Blotting Procedure and Total Mouth Hygiene. Osseo, WI: PHB, 1972. 10. Print.

57 Nield-Gehrig, Jill S., and Donald E. Willmann. Foundations of Periodontics for the Dental Hygenist. Philadelphia: Lippincott Williams & Wilkins, 2003. 262. Print.

58 Scannapieco, Frank A. Treatment of Periodontal Disease. Philadelphia, PA: W.B. Saunders, 2010. Chapter 1. Print.

59 Jan De Boever and Annemarie De Boever (2004) Occlusion and clinical practice. An evidence based approach. Chapter: Occlusion and Periodontal Health p.83-91 <https://www.elsevierhealth.com/media/us/samplechapters/ 780702026669/ 9780702026669.pdf>

60 Ibid.

61 Williams, Louisa. "From Attention Deficit to Stress Apnea. The Serious Consequences of Dental Denformities." Wise Traditions in Food, Farming and the Healing Arts. The Weston A Price Foundation. 10.3 (2009); 19-26. Print.

62 Broadbent, Jm, Kb Williams, Wm Thomson, and Sm Williams. "Dental Restorations: A Risk Factor for Periodontal Attachment Loss?" *Primary Dental Care* 14.1 (2007): 33. Web.

63 Discussion with expert cranial therapist and cranially trained dentist.

64 As taught by Dr. Gerald Smith, ICNR.COM

65 Munro-Hall, Graeme. Toxic Dentistry Exposed. 74-82. Print.

66 Gammal, Robert. "Foci of Infection." Web. 19 Dec. 2014. <http://www.robertgammal.com/RCT/FocusOnFoci.html>.

67 Smith, Gerald. "Dental, Rheumatoid Arthritis Connection." Dental, Rheumatoid Arthritis Connection. N.p., n.d. Web. 13 Nov. 2014.

68 Munro-Hall Clinic. www.munro-hallclinic.co.uk

69 GB4000 frequency machine based on Rife technology

70 Munro-Hall, Graeme. Toxic Dentistry Exposed. 74-82. Print.

71 Munro-Hall Dental Clinic, <www.munro-hallclinic.co.uk>

72 Robbins, Wendy. "Guide to Diluting Essential Oils." Guide to Diluting Essential Oils. N.p., n.d. Web. 04 Jan. 2015. <http://www.aromaweb.com/articles/dilutingessentialoils.asp>.

73 Betty, Crunchy. "21 Things You Should Know About Using Essential Oils." <http://www.crunchybetty.com/21-things-you-should-know-about-essential-oils>.

74 Nishida, M. Grossi, SG. et al. "Calcium and the risk for periodontal disease." *Journal of Periodontology*. 71.7 (2000): 66. Print

75 Manhart, Mark J. "Salivary and Blood Calcium Response to the Calcium Method of Periodontal Therapy." Calcium Therapy Institute. 1982. Web. <http://www.calciumtherapy.com/salivary-and-blood-calcium/>

76 Manhart, Mark J. " What is Calcium Therapy? " Calcium Therapy Institute. Web. < http://www.calciumtherapy.com/calcium-therapy/>

77 Waters, John. "Correctable Systemic Disorders Indicated by Presence of Salivary Calculus." Correctable Systemic Disorders Indicated by Presence of Salivary Calculus. N.p., n.d. Web. 17 Oct. 2014. <https://www.seleneriverpress.com/historical-archives/all-archive-articles/166-correctable-systemic-disorders-indicated-by-presence-of-salivary-calculus>.

78 Ravald, Nils, and Carin Starkhammar Johansson. "Tooth Loss in Periodontally Treated Patients. A Long-term Study of Periodontal Disease and Root Caries." Journal of Clinical Periodontology 39.1 (2012): 73-79. Web.

79 Page, Melvin E. Degeneration, Regeneration. St. Petersburg, FL: Biochemical Research Foundation, 1949. 91. Print.

80 "Curing Gum Disease and Cavities Naturally" March 21, 2013. Web. 27 Aug. 2014. <http://www.soultravelers3.com/2013/03/curing-gum-disease-and-cavities-naturally.html>.

Chapter 10

1 "Gum Disease—O Nara." Gum Disease--O Nara. N.p., n.d. Web. 20 Oct. 2014. <http://www.whale.to/d/nara.html>.
2 "Why Can't You Lose Weight? Ask the Guy Who Made Pepsodent a Smash." Slate Magazine. N.p., n.d. Web. 28 Oct. 2014. <http://www.slate.com/articles/arts/culturebox/2012/02/an_excerpt_from_charles_duhigg_s_the_power_of_habit_.html>.
3 France Lavoie, DH, and other authors. Evaluation of Toothpastes and of the Variables." CANADIAN JOURNAL OF DENTAL HYGIENE 41.1 (2007): 44. Web.
4 Bass, Charles C., and Foster Matthew Johns. Alveolodental Pyorrhea. Philadelphia: Saunders, 1915. 152. Print.
5 Hunter, M.l., M. Addy, M.j. Pickles, and A. Joiner. "The Role of Toothpastes and Toothbrushes in the Aetiology of Tooth Wear." International Dental Journal 52.S5 (2002): 399-405. Web.
6 Khocht, Ahmed, Gary Simon, Philip Person, and Joseph L. Denepitiya. "Gingival Recession in Relation to History of Hard Toothbrush Use." Journal of Periodontology 64.9 (1993): 900-05. Web.
7 Hawkins, H. F. "A Rational Technique for the Control of Caries and Systemic Pyorrhea." Journal of Dental Research 11.2 (1931): 206.
8 Bathla, Shalu. Periodontics Revisited. New Delhi: Jaypee Brothers Medical, 2011. 270. Print.
9 "U.S. Army Public Health Command" <http://phc.amedd.army.mil/PHC%20Resource%20Library/Chooseyourweapon-toothbrush-Mar10.pdf>
10 Christopher, John. "Echinacea, Echinacea Angustifolia; (Compositae)." Echinacea, Echinacea Angustifolia; (Compositae). N.p., n.d. Web. 30 Oct. 2014. <http://online.snh.cc/files/2100/HTML/100hs_echinacea__echinacea_angustifolia.htm>.
11 Christopher, John. "Golden Seal, Hydrastis Canadensis; (Ranunculaceae)." Golden Seal, Hydrastis Canadensis; (Ranunculaceae). N.p., n.d. Web. 30 Oct. 2014. <http://online.snh.cc/files/2100/HTML/100hs_golden_seal__hydrastis_canadensis.htm>.
12 Christopher, John. "MYRRH or GUM MYRRH Commiphora Myrrha; C. Molmol; Balsamodendron Myrrha; BURSERACEAE)." MYRRH or GUM MYRRH Commiphora Myrrha; C. Molmol; Balsamodendron Myrrha; BURSERACEAE). N.p., n.d. Web. 30 Oct. 2014. <http://online.snh.cc/files/2100/HTML/snh_myrrh.htm>.
13 Various sites posting, Abrasiveness Index of Common Toothpastes. I could not locate the original source.
14 Rasines, Graciela. "The Use of Interdental Brushes along with Toothbrushing Removes Most Plaque." Evidence-Based Dentistry 10.3 (2009): 74.
15 Fischman, Stuart L. "The History of Oral Hygiene Products: How Far Have We Come in 6000 Years?" Periodontology 2000 15.1 (1997): 7-14. Web.
16 Breiner, Mark A.. *Whole-Body Dentistry: Discover The Missing Piece To Better Health.* 1 ed. Fairfield: Quantum Health Press, 1999. Print.
17 Hawkins, Harold F. Applied Nutrition. Gardena, Cal.: Institute Pr., 1940. 9. Print.
18 Hawkins, Harold F. Applied Nutrition. Gardena, Cal.: Institute Pr., 1940. 10. Print.
19 Genco, Robert J., and Ray C. Williams. Periodontal Disease and Overall Health: A Clinician's Guide. Yardley, PA: Professional Audience Communications, 2010. 8-9. Print.
20 Ibid.
21 Ibid.
22 Nsaid/fluoride Periodontal Compositions. Sepracor Inc, assignee. Patent US 5807541 A. 15 Sept. 1998. Print.
23 Phillips, Joseph E. Acquiring and Maintaining Oral Health: Through the Blotting Procedure and Total Mouth Hygiene. Osseo, WI: PHB, 1972. 9. Print.
24 Ibid., 6.
25 Ibid.
26 Ibid.
27 Ibid., 10.

INDEX

Made in the USA
Las Vegas, NV
20 February 2024